Intercollegiate MRCS

Clinical Problem Solving EMQS

Volume 2

Charles H. Knowles BChir PhD FRCS
SpR and Clinical Lecturer in Academic Surgery
Barts and The London
Queen Mary's School of Medicine and Dentistry
University of London

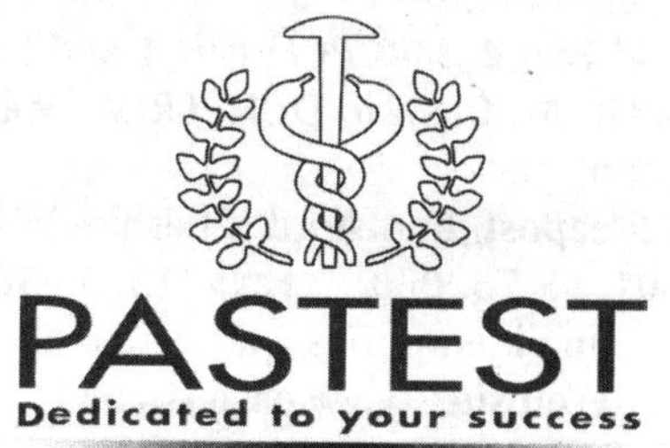

Egerton Court
Parkgate Estate
Knutsford
Cheshire WA16 8DX

Telephone: 01565 752000

A percentage of the questions were previously published in *MRCS System Modules: The Complete Test* and *MRCS Core Modules: The Complete Test.*

First edition 2005
ISBN 1 904627 404
ISBN 978 1904627 40 1

A catalogue record for this book is available from the British Library.

Typeset by Type Study, Scarborough, North Yorkshire
Printed by Alden Group Limited, Oxfordshire

CONTENTS

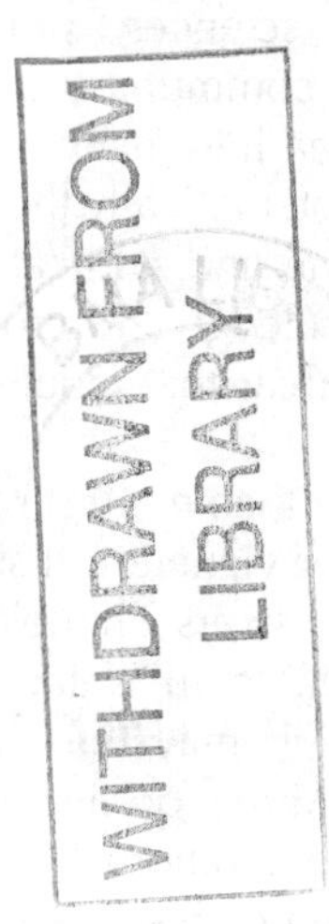

PREFACE

In medical education, many techniques have been introduced to extend the area covered by a single examination and to standardise the marking system. This text is devoted to the extended matching question (EMQ), a newer technique that is now being used alongside the multiple choice question (MCQ) and other methods of examination. It has been used in North America since the 1990s, and after its introduction into the UK by the Royal College of General Practitioners for the MRCGP examination, it has gained favour with a number of the Royal Colleges and Medical Schools. EMQs are able to cover a wide area of the curriculum and assess the candidate's knowledge of clinically relevant information. They also go beyond the recall of simple factual information, and assess the candidate's ability to draw from realistic, often existing, clinical problems.

The EMQ has now become firmly established in the armamentarium available to the surgical examiner and the Royal Colleges of Great Britain and Ireland have adopted the format to run alongside MCQs in the Inter-collegiate MRCS examination. Whilst basic sciences will continue to be largely examined in an MCQ format, the Clinical Problem Solving (Part 2) section of the examination will incorporate a significant number of EMQs. This book is primarily intended for candidates sitting this examination. The extended matching questions have been specifically structured to reflect the new changes in the syllabus of the Surgical Royal Colleges of Great Britain and Ireland. The current syllabus (May 2004) is divided into four sections: basic sciences, principles of surgery in general, surgical specialties and communication skills. These four broad categories are further subdivided into many sections. This book follows this syllabus and aims to cover systematically the two main clinical sections, ie principles of surgery in general and surgical specialties. The goal of such a book is to help assess knowledge and provide an adjunct to reading, in addition to alerting one to areas that require further study.

Each EMQ has a theme, a list of options, an introductory statement and a series of stems or vignettes. It should be stressed that all options within a list are feasible answers. I hope therefore that the lists contained herein will also prove valuable in isolation, eg differential diagnoses of common symptoms/signs. It may thus be pertinent to study these lists, perhaps identifying the three or five commonest or most important items for clinicals/vivas. In addition, the answers and explanations for each question are more detailed than some other texts and will hopefully provide many further key facts for the candidate.

Finally, I hope that this book will not be restricted only to candidates sitting the MRCS examination but will be of use also to the more ambitious Final Year medical student.

Charles H. Knowles (Editor)

CONTRIBUTORS

Editor:

Charles H Knowles BChir PhD FRCS, SpR and Clinical Lecturer in Academic Surgery, Barts and The London, Queen Mary's School of Medicine and Dentistry

Contributors:

Marc A Gladman MB BS MRCOG MRCS (Eng), Specialist Registrar in General Surgery, Barts and The London, Queen Mary's School of Medicine and Dentistry

Julia Dench MRCS (Eng), Colorectal Research Fellow, The Royal London Hospital

Toby M Hammond MB ChB MRCS (Eng), Colorectal Research Fellow, Barts and The London, Queen Mary's School of Medicine and Dentistry

Narinder Kullar MB BS MRCS, Honorary Research Fellow, Barts and The London, Queen Mary's School of Medicine and Dentistry

Mayoni L Gooneratne BSc (Hons) MB BS MRCS, Colorectal Research Fellow, Barts and The London, Queen Mary's School of Medicine and Dentistry

EXAMINATION TECHNIQUE

The written section of the new Intercollegiate Membership examination of the Surgical Royal Colleges of Great Britain and Ireland has undergone recent revision (2004) and now comprises two written papers: Part 1 for Applied Basic Sciences (ABS) and Part 2 for Clinical Problem Solving (CPS). The Part 1 ABS paper consists of multiple true false questions only. Candidates are allowed 3 hours for the paper. The Part 2 CPS consists of extended matching questions only and is presently 2½ hours in length but from April 2005 will last 3 hours.

Pacing yourself accurately during the examination to finish on time, or with time to spare, is essential. There are two common mistakes which cause good candidates to fail the MRCS written examinations. These are neglecting to read the directions and questions carefully enough and failing to fill in the computer answer card properly. You must read the instructions given to candidates at the beginning of each section of the paper to ensure that you complete the answer sheet correctly.

You must also decide on a strategy to follow with regard to marking your answer sheet. The answer sheet is read by an automatic document reader and transfers the information to a computer. It is critical that the answer sheet is filled in clearly and accurately using the pencils provided. Failure to fill in your name and your examination correctly could result in the rejection of your paper.

Some candidates mark their answers directly onto the computer sheet as they go through the questions, others prefer to make a note of their answers on the question paper, and reserve time at the end to transfer their answers onto the computer sheet. If you choose the first method, there is a chance that you may decide to change your answer after a second reading. If you do change your answer on the computer sheet, you must ensure that your original is thoroughly erased. If you choose the second method, make sure that you allow enough time to transfer your answers methodically onto the computer sheet, as rushing at this stage could introduce some costly mistakes. You will find it less confusing if you transfer your marks after you have completed each section of the examination. You must ensure that you have left sufficient time to transfer your marks from the question paper to the answer sheet. You should also be aware that no additional time will be given at the end of the examination to allow you to transfer your marks.

If you find that you have time left at the end of the examination, there can be a temptation to re-read your answers time and time again, so that even those that seemed straightforward will start to look less convincing. In this situation, first thoughts are usually best, don't alter your initial answers unless you are sure.

You must also ensure that you read the question (both stem and items) carefully. Regard each item as being independent of every other item, each referring to a specific quantum of knowledge. For the CPS section, it is important to choose the *most likely* answer as there may be more than one 'correct' answer. For every correct answer you will gain a mark (+1). Marks will not be deducted for a wrong answer. Equally, you will not gain a mark if you mark both true and false.

For this reason you should answer evey question as you have nothing to lose. If you do not know the answer to a question, you should make an educated guess – you may well get the answer right and gain a mark.

If you feel that you need to spend more time puzzling over a question, leave it and, if you have time, return to it. Make sure you have collected all the marks you can before you come back to any difficult questions.

Multiple choice questions are not designed to trick you or confuse you, they are designed to test your knowledge of medicine. Accept each question at face value.

The aim of this book is to give you practice and therefore aid revision for the Part 2 CPS paper. The broad range of questions is to test your knowledge on specific subjects.

Working through the questions in this book will help you to identify your weak subject areas. In the last few weeks before the exam it will be important for you to avoid minor unimportant areas and concentrate on the most important subject areas covered in the exam.

ABBREVIATIONS

AAA	abdominal aortic aneurysm
ABPI	arterial blood pressure index
ACE	angiotensin-converting enzyme
ACTH	adrenocorticotropic hormone
ADH	antidiuretic hormone
α-FP	alpha-fetoprotein
AIDS	acquired immunodeficiency syndrome
ASD	atrial septal defect
AXR	abdominal X-ray
BP	blood pressure
C1 etc. segment	cervical spinal segment
CBD	common bile duct
CEA	carcinoembryonic antigen
CIN	cervical intraepithelial neoplasia
CMF	cyclophosphamide, methotrexate and 5-FU (regimen)
CNS	central nervous system
COPD	chronic obstructive pulmonary disease
CRP	C-reactive protein
CSF	cerebrospinal fluid
CT	computed tomography
CVA	cerebral vascular accident
CXR	chest X-ray
DMSA	dimercaptosuccinic acid
DTPA	diethylene triamine pentacetic acid
DVT	deep venous thrombosis
ECG	electrocardiogram
ERCP	endoscopic retrograde cholangiopancreatography
ESR	erythrocyte sedimentation ratio
ESWL	extracorporeal shock wave lithotripsy
EUA	examination under anaesthesia
FAP	familial adenomatous polyposis
FBC	full blood count
GCS	Glasgow coma scale
GI	gastrointestinal
GP	general practitioner
β-hCG	human chorionic gonadotrophin
HIV	human immunodeficiency virus
HLA	human leukocyte antigen
IV	intravenous
IVU	intravenous urogram
JVP	jugular venous pressure

KUB	kidney and upper bladder
MEN	multiple endocrine neoplasia
MI	myocardial infarction
MRA	magnetic resonance angiography
MRI	magnetic resonance imaging
MRSA	methicillin-resistant *Staphylococcus aureus*
MSU	mid-stream urine system
NEC	necrotising enterocolitis
NSAID	non-specific anti-inflammatory drug
PCNL	percutaneous nephrolithotomy
Pco_2	partial pressure of carbon dioxide
PDS	polydioxanone
PE	pulmonary embolism
Po_2	partial pressure of oxygen
PP	pulse pressure
PSA	prostatic specific antigen
PTFE	polytetrafluoroethylene
PUJ	pelvi-ureteric junction
RTA	road traffic accident
RUQ	right upper quadrant
SCC	squamous-cell carcinoma
SFA	superficial femoral artery
SLR	straight leg raise
SMA	superior mesenteric artery
T1 etc. segment	thoracic spinal segment
TB	tuberculosis
TEDS	thromboembolic deterrent stockings
TIA	transient ischaemic attack
TPA	tissue plasminogen activator
TURBT	transurethral resection of bladder tumour
TURP	transurethral resection of the prostate
UTI	urinary tract infection
VIP	vasoactive intestinal peptide
VSD	ventricular septal defect
WBC	white blood cells
WCC	white cell count

QUESTIONS

QUESTIONS

PRINCIPLES OF SURGERY IN GENERAL

Peri-operative care

1 THEME: PRE-OPERATIVE FITNESS FOR SURGERY

A Electrocardiogram only
B Electrocardiogram and Urea & Electrolytes
C Full blood count (FBC) only
D FBC and electrocardiogram
E FBC, electrocardiogram and Urea & Electrolytes
F FBC, electrocardiogram, Urea & Electrolytes and Chest X-ray
G FBC, electrocardiogram, Urea & Electrolytes, Chest X-ray and Lung Function Tests
H FBC and Urea & Electrolytes
I No investigation required
J Urea & Electrolytes only

From the list above pick the single most appropriate answer containing the obligatory tests required for the following clinical scenarios. The items may be used once, more than once, or not at all.

☐ **1** A 37-year-old man who is ASA (American Society of Anaesthesiologists) Grade 1 is due to undergo a minor (Grade 1) procedure under general anaesthetic.

☐ **2** A 48-year-old woman who is ASA Grade 2 secondary to cardiovascular disease requires a major (Grade 3) operation.

☐ **3** An 83-year-old woman who is ASA Grade 2 secondary to renal disease requires a major, complex (Grade 4) procedure.

2 THEME: CONSENT FOR SURGERY

A Advance refusal
B Battery
C Best interests (treatment in) under common law
D Consent for medical research
E Implied consent (assent)
F Informed consent
G Negligence
H Parental consent
I Treatment under the Mental Health Act
J Ward of court

The following descriptions all refer to issues concerning informed consent for surgery. Please select the most appropriate term from the above list. The items may be used once, more than once, or not at all.

☐ **1** A 33-year-old glamour model with severe endometriosis underwent an abdominal hysterectomy/adhesiolysis for chronic pelvic pain. At the time of laparotomy, the uterus was found to be densely adherent to the rectum. The surgeon proceeded with the operation, resulting in a rectal perforation requiring repair and formation of a colostomy. Legal action is taken by the patient against the gynaecologist.

☐ **2** A 63-year-old man underwent a laparoscopic cholecystectomy for symptomatic gallstone disease having previously had surgery for a perforated duodenal ulcer many years previously. Following a difficult procedure requiring laparoscopic adhesiolysis, the patient developed signs of an acute abdomen on the second post-operative day requiring laparotomy and small bowel resection for two perforations which had led to peritonitis. He had a stormy post-operative course on the Intensive Care Unit and eventually was left with a troublesome enterocutaneous fistula requiring further surgery. It is alleged subsequently that during consent, no mention was made of the risk of inadvertent injury to other structures such as bowel.

☐ **3** A 40-year-old women attends the colorectal outpatient clinic with rectal bleeding. Following history-taking and abdominal examination, the attending coloproctologist performed a rectal examination and proctosigmoidoscopy, the latter of which proved uncomfortable for the patient. The surgeon is surprised to find himself some time later responding to a complaint that the patient said she had not consented to the examination.

☐ **4** A 23-year-old student suffering from a bipolar disorder attempts suicide by jumping in front of a train. He suffers bilateral pneumothoraces and a flail chest. On the ward, he attempts to remove his chest drains and essential oxygen therapy. He is currently under a section 2.

3 THEME: LOCAL ANAESTHETICS: TYPES & DOSAGES

A	9 ml	F	28 ml
B	12 ml	G	56 ml
C	18 ml	H	60 ml
D	21 ml	I	84 ml
E	27 ml	J	140 ml

The following scenarios all refer to issues concerning local anaesthesia. Please select the most appropriate answer from the above list. The items may be used once, more than once, or not at all.

☐ **1** You are asked to infiltrate a surgical wound with 0.25% bupivacaine. Select the maximum safe volume that can be used. The patient weighs 70 kg.

☐ **2** A 6-year-old child weighing 20 kg is scheduled for hernia repair. The anaesthetist wishes to supplement general anaesthesia with an ilioinguinal nerve block. He decides to use 0.5% lidocaine with adrenaline. Select the appropriate safe volume to be administered.

☐ **3** A 72-year-old patient weighing 60 kg requires intravenous regional anaesthesia (a Bier's block) of the upper limb before manipulation of a displaced Colles' fracture. Select the maximum safe volume of the anaesthetic agent of choice (concentration 2%).

4 THEME: GENERAL ANAESTHETIC AGENTS

A	Atracurium	G	Isoflurane
B	Dantrolene sodium	H	Neostigmine
C	Enflurane	I	Nitrous oxide
D	Etomidate	J	Propofol
E	Glycopyrronium	K	Suxamethonium
F	Halothane	L	Thiopentone sodium

The above are all types of general anaesthetic agents. Indicate the most appropriate drug from the list that fits the clinical scenarios below. The items may be used once, more than once, or not at all.

☐ **1** A 29-year-old man, involved in a serious road traffic accident, requires an urgent laparotomy. Rapid sequence induction is undertaken by the anaesthetic Senior House Officer. It is noted post-operatively that the patient appears to take longer than usual to begin self-ventilating.

☐ **2** A 35-year-old woman undergoing elective laparoscopy is induced using an intravenous anaesthetic agent. Her systolic blood pressure rapidly drops to 70 mmHg and a wheeze is audible in the anaesthetic room.

☐ **3** A previously well, 50-year-old woman is noted in the post-operative period to develop progressive jaundice. She was maintained on an inhalational anaesthetic agent for an open reduction and internal fixation of an ankle fracture. Liver function tests: bilirubin, 190; aspartate aminotransferase (AST), 345; alanine aminotransferase (ALP), 120; γ-glutamyltransferase, 115.

☐ **4** An extreme sportsman who has recently returned from a diving trip to Egypt is awaiting elective repair of his right inguinal hernia. What agent should be avoided in his general anaesthetic regimen?

5 THEME: COAGULATION DISORDERS

A Antithrombin III deficiency
B Disseminated intravascular coagulation (DIC)
C Factor V Leiden deficiency
D Haemophilia A
E Haemophilia B
F Idiopathic thrombocytopenia purpura (ITP)
G Protein C deficiency
H Protein S deficiency
I Thrombasthenia (Glanzmann's disease)
J Thrombocytosis
K Vitamin K deficiency
L Von Willebrand's disease

The terms above all refer to types of coagulation disorders. Please select the most appropriate term from this list for the scenarios below. The items may be used once, more than once, or not at all.

☐ **1** A 45-year-old woman, with a vague history of pulmonary embolism (PE), has developed a deep vein thrombosis (DVT) following a laparoscopic cholecystectomy. She is currently taking warfarin but has begun to notice multiple areas of skin necrosis on her body.

☐ **2** A 34-year-old man undergoes a total colectomy with ileostomy for severe refractory ulcerative colitis. He develops a post-operative septicaemia and is transferred to the Intensive Care Unit where intravenous antibiotic therapy is commenced. Nine days following transfer, he is noted to develop purpura and begins oozing from venepuncture sites. There is no personal or family history of a bleeding tendency. Haemoglobin, 9.9; white cell count, 6.3; platelets, 300; prothrombin time 26 s, activated partial thromboplastin time 60 s, thrombin time 18 s, bleeding time 5 min.

☐ **3** A male infant suffers from a profuse post-circumcision haemorrhage and his mother mentions that her brother had a clotting problem that requires regular Factor VIII infusions.

6 THEME: TYPES OF ANAEMIA

A Aplastic anaemia
B Autoimmune haemolytic anaemia
C Chronic disease
D Folate deficiency
E Haemorrhage
F Hereditary spherocytosis
G Hypersplenism
H Iron deficiency
I Microangiopathic haemolytic anaemia
J Pernicious anaemia
K Sickle cell anaemia
L Sideroblastic anaemia
M Thalassaemia
N Vitamin B_{12} deficiency

The following are descriptions of patients' symptoms with types of surgically important anaemia. Please select the most appropriate diagnosis from the list. The items may be used once, more than once, or not at all.

☐ **1** A 47-year-old Afro-Caribbean man presents with fatigue, diarrhoea and steatorrhoea 12-weeks after ileal resection for isolated Crohn's disease. Examination is unremarkable. Full blood count reveals haemoglobin 8.6 g/dl and mean corpuscular volume 110 fl.

☐ **2** A 42-year-old Caucasian woman presents to The Emergency Department with jaundice and right upper quadrant abdominal pain; her past medical history includes systemic lupus erythematosis. Examination confirms clinical jaundice and reveals moderate splenomegaly. Blood tests reveal haemoglobin 9.0 g/dl and mean corpuscular volume 90 fl. She has a positive direct Coombs' test.

☐ **3** A 74-year-old Afro-Caribbean man presents with lethargy, weight loss and right-sided abdominal pain. Examination is unremarkable. Blood tests reveal haemoglobin 10.0 g/dl and mean corpuscular volume 72 fl.

7 THEME: BLOOD TRANSFUSION COMPLICATIONS

A Air embolism
B Allergic reaction
C Bacterial contamination
D Cannulation site thrombophlebitis
E Circulatory overload
F Delayed haemolytic transfusion reaction
G Graft-versus-host disease
H Hyperkalaemia
I Hypocalcaemia
J Hypothermia
K Immediate haemolytic transfusion reaction
L Immunosuppression
M Iron overload
N Non-haemolytic febrile transfusion reaction
O Post-transfusion purpura
P Transfusion-related acute lung injury (TRALI)
Q Transfusion-transmitted infection
R Urticaria

The following patients all have complications of blood transfusion. Please select the most appropriate cause or description from the above list. The items may be used once, more than once, or not at all.

☐ **1** You are called to see a 35-year-old multiparous woman on your surgical ward who, 6 days after an intra-operative blood transfusion, is complaining of nose bleeds and sacral bruising. A coagulation screen is normal. Her platelet count is 28×10^9/litre.

☐ **2** A 40-year-old man, with no history of pulmonary disease, develops acute dyspnoea within 16 h of receiving a whole blood transfusion. His oxygen saturations on air are 90%. Arterial blood gas $p_A(O_2)$ is 9.0 kPa. A chest X-ray shows patchy shadowing in both lung fields.

☐ **3** A 24-year-old female pedestrian is admitted unconscious to the Intensive Care Unit after a hit-and-run accident. She has been appropriately assessed and managed for her injuries. A blood transfusion has just been commenced. Having remained previously stable, you now notice that she is spiking a temperature of 39.5 °C, her blood pressure is 100/60 mmHg, and she is bleeding profusely through her wound dressings and oozing blood around her venepuncture sites. Her catheter contains dark urine that is dipstick positive for haemoglobinuria.

☐ **4** A 26-year-old Afro-Caribbean woman presents to her general practitioner (GP) with symptoms of lethargy and weight gain. She is known to have sickle cell anaemia and, because of multiple painful crises, has required regular blood transfusions. Blood tests requested by her GP show: thyroid-stimulating hormone 9 μmol/litre, free thyroxine 7 pmol/litre, calcium 2.15 mmol/litre. Further investigations reveal poor cardiac function.

Post-operative management and critical care

8 THEME: ARTERIAL BLOOD GASES

A Compensated metabolic acidosis
B Compensated metabolic alkalosis
C Compensated respiratory acidosis
D Compensated respiratory alkalosis
E Metabolic acidosis and increased anion gap
F Metabolic acidosis and normal anion gap
G Metabolic alkalosis
H Respiratory acidosis
I Respiratory alkalosis

The following are descriptions of patients' symptoms with arterial blood gas abnormalities. Please select the most appropriate interpretation of the arterial blood gases from the list. The items may be used once, more than once, or not at all.

☐ **1** A 57-year-old man undergoes an oesophagogastrectomy for low oesophageal carcinoma; the operation lasts 4 h. Six hours post-operatively his arterial blood gases are: pH 7.31, $p_A(O_2)$ 11.6 kPa, $p_A(CO_2)$ 4.7 kPa, base excess −5 mmol/litre; serum blood results are: Na^+ 138 mmol/litre, K^+ 4.0 mmol/litre, urea 11.0 mmol/litre, creatinine 100 μmol/litre, Cl^- 100 mmol/litre, HCO_3^- 22 mmol/litre.

☐ **2** A 64-year-old man undergoes an anterior resection for rectal carcinoma. On day 7 post-operation his arterial blood gases are: pH 7.35, $p_A(O_2)$ 10.2 kPa, $p_A(CO_2)$ 2.5 kPa, base excess −8 mmol/litre; serum blood results are: Na^+ 138 mmol/litre, K^+ 4.0 mmol/litre, urea 14.0 mmol/litre, creatinine 100 μmol/litre, Cl^- 100 mmol/litre, HCO_3^- 16 mmol/litre. He has become increasingly unwell for the past 2 days.

☐ **3** A 45-year-old woman presents to The Emergency Department with a 3-day history of upper abdominal pain and profuse vomiting. Her arterial blood gases are: pH 7.45, $p_A(O_2)$ 12.2 kPa, $p_A(CO_2)$ 7.1 kPa, base excess +10 mmol/litre; serum blood results are: Na^+ 138 mmol/litre, K^+ 3.0 mmol/litre, urea 14.0 mmol/litre, creatinine 100 µmol/litre, Cl^- 90 mmol/litre, HCO_3^- 40 mmol/litre.

☐ **4** A 21-year-old woman undergoes an emergency splenectomy for a trauma; her pain is poorly controlled post-operation. On day 2 post-operation her arterial blood gases are: pH 7.32, $p_A(O_2)$ 8.4 kPa, $p_A(CO_2)$ 7.4 kPa, base excess −2 mmol/litre; serum blood results are: Na^+ 138 mmol/litre, K^+ 3.0 mmol/litre, urea 2.0 mmol/litre, creatinine 90 µmol/litre, Cl^- 100 mmol/litre, HCO_3^- 28 mmol/litre.

9 THEME: POST-OPERATIVE HYPOXIA

A	Adult respiratory distress syndrome	F	Opiate overdose
B	Basal atelectasis	G	Pleural effusion
C	Bronchospasm	H	Pneumonia
D	Cardiogenic pulmonary oedema	I	Pneumothorax
E	Lobar collapse	J	Pulmonary embolism
		K	Upper airway obstruction

The following are descriptions of patients with post-operative hypoxia. Please select the most appropriate diagnosis from the above list. The items may be used once, more than once, or not at all.

☐ **1** A 62-year-old woman undergoes a sigmoid colectomy for left-sided colonic carcinoma. She is given an epidural for pain relief, but this becomes dislodged. On day 1 post-operation she is dyspnoeic with a rapid pulse and mild pyrexia; auscultation reveals reduced breath sounds at the left base. Arterial blood gases are: pH 7.35, $p_A(O_2)$ 9.6 kPa, $p_A(CO_2)$ 5.0 kPa. She has a non-productive cough.

☐ **2** A 74-year-old man with a previous history of ischaemic heart disease undergoes an anterior resection for rectal carcinoma. On day 4 post-operation he is severely dyspnoeic, tachypnoeic but apyrexial; auscultation reveals bilateral fine crepitations. Arterial blood gases are: pH 7.35, $p_A(O_2)$ 8.0 kPa, $p_A(CO_2)$ 5.5 kPa.

☐ **3** A 59-year-old man undergoes a palliative bypass of an unresectable gastric carcinoma. Several days later he is dyspnoeic, mildly tachycardic and apyrexial; auscultation reveals absent breath sounds at the left base and decreased left-sided vocal resonance. Arterial blood gases are: pH 7.37, $p_A(O_2)$ 10.1 kPa, $p_A(CO_2)$ 6.0 kPa. His serum albumin is 20 g/litre.

☐ **4** A 43-year-old woman is being managed for severe acute pancreatitis. Over the past 48 h she has become increasingly dyspnoeic and tachycardic; auscultation reveals bilateral fine crepitations. Arterial blood gases are: pH 7.37, $p_A(O_2)$ 8.2 kPa, $p_A(CO_2)$ 4.9 kPa. Chest radiology shows bilateral diffuse infiltrates.

10 THEME: POST-OPERATIVE PYREXIA

A	Abdominal ultrasound scan	H	CT thorax
B	Abdominal X-ray	I	Duplex ultrasound scan
C	Arterial blood gases	J	Exploratory laparotomy
D	Barium enema	K	Joint aspiration and culture
E	Blood cultures	L	Urine culture
F	Chest X-ray	M	Venography
G	Computed tomography (CT) abdomen	N	Water-soluble contrast enema
		O	Wound swab

The following are descriptions of patients' symptoms with post-operative pyrexia. Please select the most appropriate investigation from the list. The items may be used once, more than once, or not at all.

☐ **1** A 74-year-old man undergoes an oesophagogastrectomy for carcinoma. He has an epidural at the level of the seventh thoracic vertebra. On day 1 post-operation he develops a temperature of 37.8 °C.

☐ **2** A 42-year-old woman undergoes an uncomplicated laparoscopic cholecystectomy. She is discharged the following day. She returns to casualty 4 days later with intermittent fever, sweats and abdominal pain. Examination reveals a temperature of 38.5 °C and tenderness in the right upper quadrant.

☐ **3** A 60-year-old man undergoes a right total knee replacement. On day 7 post-operation the patient develops pain and swelling along the right thigh. Examination reveals a temperature of 39 °C, tenderness along the medial aspect of the affected thigh and pitting oedema.

☐ **4** A 54-year-old lady undergoes an anterior resection for rectal carcinoma. On day 5 post-operation she develops abdominal pain. On examination she has a temperature of 38.7 °C, a pulse rate of 128/min and the abdomen is peritonitic.

11 THEME: POST-OPERATIVE OLIGURIA

A Acute renal failure
B Cardiogenic shock
C Covert haemorrhage
D Increased ADH secretion
E Obstructed urinary catheter
F Overt haemorrhage
G Sepsis
H Severe diarrhoea
I Severe vomiting
J Third space loss
K Urinary retention

The above are all causes of post-operative oliguria. For the following scenarios please pick the most appropriate answer from the list. Each item may be used once, more than once, or not at all.

☐ **1** A 64-year-old man has undergone surgery for repair of his 6.5-cm abdominal aortic aneurysm. He is recovering on the High Dependency Unit when the nurses call you to inform you that he has passed only 5–10 ml/hr of urine for the past 6 h, despite catheter flushing. On examination you note that his abdomen is not distended, his blood pressure is 130/75 mmHg; his pulse is 95/min and his central venous pressure is 12 cmH_2O. You are awaiting blood results. The operative note reveals that the origin of the aneurysm was at vertebral level L2.

☐ **2** A 60-year-old diabetic man is recovering from a left femoro-popliteal bypass. The nurses call you to let you know that he has failed to pass more than 5 ml/h of urine for the past 3 h. They have been giving him Gaviscon for 'indigestion' which has not settled. On examination you note that he is pale and sweaty. His blood pressure is 95/60 mmHg and his pulse is 98/min. The bandages covering his operative wound are minimally blood-stained and his thigh, although slightly swollen, is soft. Two fluid challenges each of 250 ml of Gelofusin fail to improve his blood pressure.

12 THEME: ENTERAL AND PARENTERAL NUTRITION

A Eating and drinking
B Elemental diet
C Feeding jejunostomy
D Fortisips/Ensure
E Low-volume, low-electrolyte feed
F Modular diet
G Nasogastric feeding
H Nasojejunal feeding
I Peptide diet
J Percutaneous endoscopic gastrostomy feeding
K Total parenteral nutrition

The above are all examples of types and routes of nutritional support. For the following statements please choose the most appropriate option from the list. Each item may be used once, more than once, or not at all.

☐ **1** The best route of early post-operative feeding following Ivor–Lewis oesophagectomy.

☐ **2** A patient with chronic renal failure managed by continuous ambulatory peritoneal dialysis requires feeding via a nasogastric tube. What is the most appropriate type of feed?

☐ **3** The best route for nutrition in a stroke patient who requires feeding for the foreseeable future (> 4 weeks).

☐ **4** A patient who has had a superior mesenteric arterial infarction is recovering post-operatively. The surgical notes state that only 95 cm of small bowel were viable at operation and a small bowel stoma was formed. The patient requires nutritional support.

☐ **5** A patient with predicted acute severe pancreatitis is transferred to the High Dependency Unit. You are asked by 'enlightened' staff to make a plan for ongoing nutritional support.

13 THEME: ANTI-EMETICS

A Cyclizine
B Metoclopramide
C Nabilone
D Ondansetron
E Prochlorperazine
F Scopolamine

The following statements describe the mechanism(s) of action of pharmaceutical agents used in the treatment of nausea and vomiting. From the list above, select the most likely anti-emetic agent. The items may be used once, more than once, or not at all.

☐ **1** A dopamine antagonist that acts almost exclusively centrally by blocking the chemoreceptor trigger zone in the area postrema.

☐ **2** An antagonist that acts on both central receptors in the area postrema and peripheral receptors on upper gastrointestinal afferent neurones.

14 THEME: SURGICAL ANALGESIA

A Aspirin
B Buprenorphine
C Celecoxib
D Co-proxamol
E Dextropropoxyphene
F Diclofenac
G Fentanyl
H Ibuprufen
I Morphine
J Naproxen
K Pethidine
L Tramadol

The following are descriptions of analgesics used to relieve post-operative pain. Please select the most appropriate analgesic from the above list. The items may be used once, more than once, or not at all.

☐ **1** A synthetic analogue of codeine with a comparatively low incidence of dependence. It produces analgesia by two mechanisms: an opioid effect, with low affinity for central μ-receptors and an enhancement of serotonergic and adrenergic pathways.

☐ **2** A prostaglandin synthesis antagonist, which acts primarily via selective inhibition of cyclo-oxygenase-2 receptors.

Surgical technique

15 THEME: SURGICAL INSTRUMENTS

A Allis forceps
B Babcock forceps
C Debakey forceps
D Dunhill clamp
E Eisenhammer retractor
F Littlewood forceps
G Lloyd Davies clamp
H Moynihan clamp
I Norfolk–Norwich retractor
J Officer forceps
K Parker–Kerr clamp
L Robert clamp
M Travers retractor

The following are descriptions of surgical instruments. Please select the most appropriate instrument from the list. The items may be used once, more than once, or not at all.

☐ **1** A 62-year-old gentleman is undergoing a Milligan–Morgan haemorrhoidectomy. Select an instrument commonly used to gain exposure.

☐ **2** A 21-year-old woman is undergoing an appendicectomy. The peritoneum has been opened and the appendix has been identified. Select the most appropriate instrument with which to enclose the tip of the appendix to facilitate its subsequent dissection.

☐ **3** A 57-year-old gentleman is undergoing a segmental colectomy. Select the instrument most commonly used to clamp the main vascular pedicles before division and ligation.

☐ **4** Select suitable dissecting forceps for performing vascular surgery.

16 THEME: SUTURE MATERIALS

A Catgut
B Dermalon/surgilon
C Dexon
D Ethibond
E Ethilon/nurolon
F Maxon
G Mersilene/Ti-cron
H Novafil
I PDS
J Prolene
K Vicryl
L Silk
M Steel wire

All the above are examples of common suture materials. Please pick the most appropriate from the list for the operative procedures below. The items may be used once, more than once, or not at all.

☐ **1** Mass closure of a laparotomy wound (using an absorbable suture).

☐ **2** Closure of a cardiac sternotomy wound.

☐ **3** Vascular anastomosis in a femoro-popliteal bypass.

☐ **4** Suture of choice for anchoring mesh in an inguinal hernia repair.

17 THEME: SURGICAL INCISIONS

A Gable
B Gridiron (or skin crease modification)
C Kocher
D Lanz
E Lateral thoracotomy
F Left paramedian
G Long midline
H Lower midline
I Median sternotomy
J Right paramedian
K Rutherford–Morrison
L Thoracoabdominal
M Transverse 'unilateral' Pfannenstiel
N Upper midline

The following are descriptions of patients requiring surgery. Please select the most appropriate incision for the required operation from the list. The items may be used once, more than once, or not at all.

☐ **1** A 72-year-old woman presents to The Emergency Department with a 1-day history of a painful lump in the left groin and vomiting. On examination she has a hard, tender, irreducible mass just below the inguinal ligament.

☐ **2** A 21-year-old man presents with a 3-day history of worsening lower right abdominal pain associated with anorexia. On examination, he is pyrexial and tachycardic. He has rebound tenderness in the right iliac fossa.

☐ **3** A 38-year-old woman has been taking regular diclofenac for relief of chronic backache. She is referred to The Emergency Department with sudden onset of upper abdominal pain. On examination she is pyrexial and tachycardic, abdominal examination reveals severe epigastric tenderness. There is a pneumoperitoneum evident on an erect chest X-ray.

18 THEME: ON-TABLE POSITIONS

A Armchair
B Lateral
C Lateral decubitus
D Lithotomy
E Lloyd Davies
F Prone
G Prone jack-knife
H Reverse Trendelenberg
I Supine
J Trendelenberg

Above is a list of positions that are employed for various surgical procedures. From the operations described below please choose the most suitable on-table position. The items may be used once, more than once, or not at all.

☐ **1** A 60-year-old man undergoing abdomino-perineal excision of the rectum.

☐ **2** A 42-year-old woman undergoing long saphenous vein high ligation, stripping and avulsions.

☐ **3** A 64-year-old woman requiring a right-sided nephrectomy for renal cell carcinoma.

☐ **4** A 35-year-old man having an arthroscopic rotator cuff repair.

19 THEME: LAPAROSCOPIC COMPLICATIONS

A Abdominal wall emphysema
B Bleeding
C Carbon dioxide embolus
D Lower limb venous thromboembolism
E Omental emphysema
F Pneumomediastinum
G Pneumothorax
H Port site hernia
I Reduced venous return
J Respiratory compromise
K Visceral injury: obstruction
L Visceral injury: perforation

The above are all descriptions of complications that may arise as a result of laparoscopic surgery. For each clinical scenario please select the most appropriate answer from the above list. The items may be used once, more than once, or not at all.

☐ **1** A 45-year-old obese man is undergoing a laparoscopic cholecystectomy. The abdomen has been rapidly insufflated with carbon dioxide. The anaesthetist alerts you to a sudden and rapid drop in blood pressure with a concomitant tachycardia. There is no evidence of intra-abdominal bleeding on inspection with the scope.

☐ **2** A 26-year-old woman returns to the ward after an exploratory laparoscopy for right iliac fossa pain. As the anaesthetic wears off she begins to complain of abdominal discomfort. On palpation you note crepitus over her abdominal wall.

☐ **3** A 51-year-old woman undergoes a difficult laparoscopic cholecystectomy. In the ensuing 48 h she develops jaundice. Liver function tests are: AP 250 mmol/litre, bilirubin 147 mmol/litre. An urgent endoscopic cholangiogram does not delineate the intra-hepatic biliary tree.

Research and management issues

20 THEME: BASIC STATISTICS (TAXONOMY)

A Analysis of variance (ANOVA)
B χ^2 test
C Correlation
D False negatives
E False positives
F Likelihood ratio
G Negative predictive value
H Positive predictive value
I Power analysis
J Regression analysis
K Sensitivity
L Specificity
M *t*-tests

The following descriptions all refer to basic statistical methods that are commonly employed in medical research. Please select the most appropriate term from the above list. The items may be used once, more than once, or not at all.

☐ **1** A method of statistical analysis used for hypothesis testing where we wish to compare proportions of categorical data.

☐ **2** In the assessment of a diagnostic test, the proportion of patients with negative test results who are correctly diagnosed.

☐ **3** This may be calculated to indicate the value of a test for increasing certainty about a positive diagnosis. It is numerically equal to the sensitivity/(1 – specificity).

21 THEME: TYPES OF SCIENTIFIC EVIDENCE

A Case–control series
B Case series
C Cohort study
D Controlled clinical trial
E Cross-sectional survey
F Experimental research paper
G Guidelines
H Meta-analysis
I Non-systematic review
J Randomised controlled trial
K Randomised double-blind controlled trial
L Systematic review
M Uncontrolled trial

The following are descriptions of types of scientific evidence. Please select the most appropriate descriptive term from the list above. The items may be used once, more than once, or not at all.

☐ **1** A statistical synthesis of the numerical results of several trials which all addressed the same question.

☐ **2** A study in which two or more groups of people are selected on the basis of differences in their exposure to a particular agent and are followed-up to observe any differences in outcome between the groups.

☐ **3** A study in which medical histories of more than one patient with a particular condition are described to illustrate one interesting aspect of the condition or treatment.

22 THEME: PRINCIPLES OF TRIAL DESIGN AND CONDUCT

A Cross-over design
B Detection bias
C Double-blinding
D Exclusion bias
E Factorial design
F Intention to treat
G Minimisation
H Null hypothesis
I Parallel group design
J Performance bias
K Power
L Selection bias
M Simple randomisation
N Single blinding
O Stratified randomisation
P Subgroup analysis
Q Type I error
R Type II error

The following are descriptions of terms used in the language of trial design. Please select the most appropriate descriptive term from the list above. The items may be used once, more than once, or not at all.

☐ **1** In hypothesis testing: the term used to describe a situation in which we fail to reject the null hypothesis when a difference is really present.

☐ **2** An erroneous influence potentially effecting the conclusions of a trial caused by systematic differences in withdrawals from the trial.

☐ **3** A method of allocation in comparative studies that provides treatment groups that are very closely similar for several variables.

23 THEME: SCIENTIFIC RESEARCH TECHNIQUES

A Cloning
B DNA fingerprinting
C DNA microarray
D DNA sequencing
E Hybridisation
F Linkage analysis
G Northern blotting
H Polymerase chain reaction
I Southern blotting
J Transfection
K Transformation
L Western blotting

The following are all brief descriptions of common molecular techniques utilised in medical research. Please select the technique which best fits each description from the above list. The items may be used once, more than once, or not at all.

☐ **1** An automated method utilising microchip technology in which the differential expression of thousands of genes can be estimated in a single experiment.

☐ **2** A method to separate and detect proteins using a denaturing sodium dodecyl sulphate–polyacrylamide gel with subsequent transfer to a membrane (usually nitrocellulose) and detection using specific antibodies.

☐ **3** An in vitro technique designed to isolate and amplify small, specific segments of DNA between 105- and 108-fold from insignificant quantities of template.

☐ **4** The transfer of a DNA fragment of interest from one organism to a self-replicating genetic element such as a bacterial plasmid, and its subsequent propagation in a foreign host cell.

24 THEME: THE LANGUAGE OF THE NEW NHS

A Audit
B Clinical Governance
C Commission for Health Improvement (CHI)
D Foundation hospitals
E Modernisation agency
F National Institute for Clinical Excellence (NICE)
G National service frameworks (NSFs)
H National targets
I NHS trusts
J Performance assessment framework (PAF)
K Primary-care groups (PCGs)
L Primary-care trusts (PCTs)
M Independent sector treatment centres (ISTCs)
N Strategic Health Authorities (SHAs)

The following are all brief descriptions of terms used within the language of the new NHS. Please select the term that best fits each description from the above list. The items may be used once, more than once, or not at all.

☐ **1** Policies that set national standards and identify key interventions for a defined service or care group.

☐ **2** New organisations bringing together groups of health workers (doctors and nurses) with community-care organisations, including social services, who are responsible for local shaping and commissioning of care.

☐ **3** A system through which NHS organisations are accountable for continuously improving the quality of their services and safeguarding high standards of care, by creating an environment in which clinical excellence will flourish.

Clinical microbiology

25 THEME: SURGICALLY IMPORTANT MICRO-ORGANISMS

A *Actinomyces*
B *Candida albicans*
C *Clostridium difficile*
D *Clostridium perfringens*
E *Corynebacterium*
F *Escherichia coli* spp.
G *Haemophilus influenzae*
H *Helicobacter pylori*
I Herpes simplex virus
J *Listeria*
K *Mycobacterium tuberculosis*
L *Neisseria meningitides*
M *Pasteurella multocida*
N *Pseudomonas aeruginosa*
O *Salmonella*
P *Staphylococcus aureus*
Q *Streptococcus pneumoniae*
R *Streptococcus pyogenes*

From the list above choose the most likely causative organism for the following clinical scenarios. The items may be used once, more than once, or not at all.

☐ **1** A 45-year-old lady develops a swinging pyrexia 4 days after an uncomplicated open inguinal hernia repair. Her wound is oozing pus from its lateral aspect.

☐ **2** A 6-year-old boy presents with a spreading cellulitis around the bite on his arm 3 days after being bitten by his family cat.

☐ **3** A 78-year-old man becomes confused and drowsy less than 48 h after transurethral resection of the prostate for benign prostatic hyperplasia. His urine is cloudy and offensive smelling.

26 THEME: COMPLICATIONS OF TUBERCULOSIS

A Bronchopneumonia
B Glomerulonephritis
C Epididymo-orchitis
D Ileitis (tabes mesenterica)
E Lupus vulgaris
F Meningitis
G Osteomyelitis
H Pericarditis
I Peritonitis
J Renal abscess
K Scrofula
L Tuberculoma

The following patients have all presented with manifestations of tuberculosis. For each, please select the most appropriate diagnosis from the above list. The items may be used once, more than once, or not at all.

☐ **1** A 39-year-old man with human immunodeficiency virus infection presents to The Emergency Department with a 3-day history of headache, malaise and vomiting. His partner has noticed that he has become increasingly confused.

☐ **2** A 53-year-old Asian man presents with difficulty of micturition followed by onset of sudden, painless urinary retention. He has been suffering from lower back pain for the last few months, which he had attributed to old age.

☐ **3** A 29-year-old homeless woman attends The Emergency Department with a large, tender mass in her supraclavicular fossa. The overlying skin appears discoloured but does not feel hot to touch.

27 THEME: APPROPRIATE ANTI-MICROBIAL THERAPY

A Acyclovir
B Cefuroxime
C Co-amoxiclav (amoxicillin + clavulanic acid)
D Co-trimoxazole (trimethoprim + sulphonamide)
E Erythromycin
F Flucloxacillin
G Gentamycin
H Imipenem
I Metronidazole
J Nystatin
K Penicillin V
L Rifampicin
M Trimethoprim
N Vancomycin

The following patients require anti-microbial therapy. For each, please select the most appropriate form of treatment from the above list. The items may be used once, more than once, or not at all.

☐ **1** A 70-year-old bronchitic man has been transferred to the Intensive Care Unit for ventilation following a complicated anterior resection. In the ensuing post-operative period, he develops signs of a chest infection. Before admission he was prescribed a course of amoxicillin for a cough by his general practitioner, and intravenous cefuroxime and metronidazole were administered at induction. A tracheal aspirate shows pus cells and a Gram-negative bacillus.

☐ **2** A 65-year-old lady develops offensive smelling, greenish-coloured loose stools following 4 days of treatment with a second-generation cephalosporin but is allergic to metronidazole.

☐ **3** A 40-year-old lady with rheumatoid arthritis presents with an acutely hot, painful, swollen knee. Emergency drainage of her joint reveals frank pus, and the primary microbiology report demonstrates polymorphs and multiple clusters of Gram-positive cocci.

28 THEME: STERILISATION AND DISINFECTION

A Alcohol
B Autoclave
C Boiling water
D Chlorhexidine-cetrimide (Savlon)
E Chlorhexidine in detergent (Hibiscrub)
F Dry heat
G Ethylene oxide
H Gamma radiation
I Glutaraldehyde
J Iodine
K Steam with formaldehyde

The above are all methods of either sterilisation or disinfection. For each of the following please select the most appropriate answer from the above list. The items may be used once, more than once, or not at all.

☐ **1** A method of sterilising sutures.

☐ **2** A method used for disinfecting endoscopes.

☐ **3** A method of sterilisation that is monitored using the Bowie–Dick test.

Emergency medicine/trauma

29 THEME: TYPES OF SHOCK

A Anaphylactic
B Cardiogenic
C Class 1 haemorrhagic
D Class 2 haemorrhagic
E Class 3 haemorrhagic
F Class 4 haemorrhagic
G Endocrine-related
H Iatrogenic
I Neurogenic
J Non-haemorrhagic hypovolaemic
K Septic
L Spinal

The following are descriptions of shock. Please select the most appropriate diagnosis from the above list. The items may be used once, more than once, or not at all.

☐ **1** A 32-year-old man is stabbed in the left side of the chest. Initial assessment reveals engorged neck veins, respiratory rate 30 breaths/min, pulse rate 120/min and blood pressure 80/40 mmHg despite attempts at fluid resuscitation; on auscultation heart sounds are muffled. His urine output has not been assessed.

☐ **2** A 72-year-old man presents with sudden onset of severe central abdominal pain radiating to the back. On examination, he is very anxious, with respiratory rate 33 breaths/min, pulse rate 120/min and blood pressure 90/40 mmHg. He has passed 15 ml of urine since he was catheterised 1 h ago. Both femoral pulses are only faintly palpable.

☐ **3** A 61-year-old man becomes acutely confused day 3 post-abdominal aortic aneurysm repair. Examination reveals temperature 38 °C, respiratory rate 36 breaths/min, pulse rate 140/min and blood pressure 90/40 mmHg despite attempts at fluid resuscitation. He has passed a negligible volume of urine since he was catheterised 1 h ago. Ironically his peripheries are warm to the touch.

30 THEME: DRUGS USED IN CRITICAL CARE

A Adenosine
B Adrenaline
C Amiodarone
D Amrinone
E Atropine
F Digoxin
G Dobutamine
H Dopamine
I Dopexamine
J Lignocaine
K Nitroglycerin
L Noradrenaline

The following are descriptions of drugs used in the management of the critically ill patient. Please select the most appropriate drug from the list. The items may be used once, more than once, or not at all.

☐ **1** A predominant β1-agonist, used to improve cardiac output in patients with myocardial failure, provided intravascular volume is satisfactory.

☐ **2** A phosphodiesterase III inhibitor; acting as both a positive inotrope and a peripheral vasodilator; it is effective in cardiogenic shock.

☐ **3** A predominant α1-agonist; the first line in patients with septic shock.

31 THEME: PRIORITIES IN IMMEDIATE TRAUMA CARE

A Airway management
B Anteroposterior chest X-ray
C Anteroposterior pelvis X-ray
D Chest drain
E Chest X-ray
F Cross-match and blood transfusion
G Intravenous access and fluid resuscitation
H Lateral cervical spine X-ray
I Pericardiocentesis
J Pneumatic anti-shock garment
K Rewarming
L Urgent neurological opinion

The following scenarios describe road traffic accidents where the patient has been brought in by ambulance with cervical spine immobilisation and 100% oxygen administered by mask. However, no other active management has been instigated. From the list above please select the most appropriate resuscitation measure with the highest priority. A measure may be chosen once, more than once, or not at all.

☐ **1** An 18-year-old motorcyclist is brought in after being thrown off his bike. He is confused and there is evidence of blood and vomit around his mouth. Vital signs: blood pressure 130/65 mmHg, pulse rate 110/min, respiratory rate 28 breaths/min.

☐ **2** A 35-year-old woman is brought to casualty after being pinned in her car following collision with a lamp post. After extrication it is apparent that she had not been wearing a seatbelt. On examination, after appropriate airway management, she demonstrates central cyanosis, distended neck veins but equal air entry with marked bruising over her anterior chest wall. Vital signs: blood pressure 80/40 mmHg, pulse rate 140/min, respiratory rate 50 breaths/min.

☐ **3** A 20-year-old man is brought in after being found under the wheel of a car. He is drowsy, aggressive but keeps complaining of abdominal and left leg pain. Vital signs: blood pressure 80/40 mmHg, pulse rate 150/min, respiratory rate 38 breaths/min.

32 THEME: MANAGEMENT DECISIONS IN TRAUMA CARE

A Abdominal X-ray
B Angiogram
C Chest drain
D Computed tomography scan
E Diagnostic peritoneal lavage
F Emergency laparotomy
G Emergency thoracotomy
H Focused Assessment Sonographically of Trauma (FAST) scan
I Fracture management
J Local wound exploration
K Resuscitation thoracotomy
L Transfer to specialist unit
M Ultrasound

In the following scenarios, each patient has undergone a primary survey, and now requires a management decision. From the list above, choose the most appropriate answer. Each item may be used once, more than once, or not at all.

☐ **1** A 38-year-old cyclist has been brought in to casualty after being knocked off his bicycle by a lorry. He was extricated from under one of the wheels, which was lying across his abdomen. He has bruising to this area and is complaining of considerable abdominal pain. He is conscious and maintaining a blood pressure of 120/70 mmHg, pulse rate 110/min and respiratory rate 20 breaths/min. A FAST scan is negative.

☐ **2** A 55-year-old gentleman has been brought in after falling 7 m off his ladder while painting the outside of his house. His fall was broken by his ladder, and he was unconscious for 3 min before being found by his wife. He has a large occipital scalp laceration that is bleeding profusely but there is no underlying skull fracture. He has, however, fractured his left ninth and tenth ribs posteriorly but has no clinical or radiographical evidence of a pneumothorax. He now has a Glasgow Coma Score of 14 with blood pressure 60/40 mmHg, pulse rate 140/min and respiratory rate 36 breaths/min. Despite aggressive fluid resuscitation, his vital signs remain the same. He has a tender left hypochondrium.

☐ **3** A 24-year-old motorcyclist is brought in after a head-on collision with a car. He was conscious on arrival but complained of pain in his chest, back and left ankle. Examination reveals a blood pressure of 100/70 mmHg, pulse rate 90/min and a respiratory rate 28 breaths/min. His ankle is deformed and painful to move. There is evidence of tracheal shift and the left hemithorax is not moving. A chest X-ray demonstrates haemopneumothorax and chest drain insertion results in immediate drainage of 1600 ml blood. Despite initial clinical improvement, the drain continues to collect fresh blood at a rate of several hundred ml per 10 min.

33 THEME: THE RED EYE

A	Acute closed-angle glaucoma	H	Hyphaema
B	Allergic conjunctivitis	I	Infective conjunctivitis
C	Anterior uveitis	J	Keratitis
D	Corneal abrasion	K	Scleritis
E	Corneal foreign body	L	Sub-conjunctival haemorrhage
F	Corneal ulceration		
G	Episcleritis		

The following patients all present complaining of a red eye. For each, please select the most appropriate diagnosis from the above list. The items may be used once, more than once, or not at all.

☐ **1** A 55-year-old woman with rheumatoid arthritis presents to The Emergency Department minors department with a 48-h history of progressively worsening pain and florid erythema to her right eye. She complains of constant watering but has not noticed any discharge. On examination she has a localised area of inflammation that is extremely tender to pressure. The injected vessels are in the deep layer of the eye.

☐ **2** A 60-year-old man attends The Emergency Department in the late evening. He describes the onset of sudden excruciating pain in his left eye associated with an episode of vomiting and 'haziness' of vision. He tells you that this has occurred twice in the past, and was relieved by going to sleep. On closer examination you note that his eye is inflamed and tender. The cornea is cloudy, and the pupil is semi-dilated and fixed in response to light.

☐ **3** A 35-year-old golfer attends the emergency eye clinic after his golfing partner accidentally caught him in the left orbit with his club. He complains of double vision and discomfort to his eye, and there is a laceration to his upper eyelid. You notice that his left eye movements are restricted during your examination, and that he has blood in the anterior chamber of his eye. Palpation reveals crepitus in the peri-orbital tissues.

☐ **4** A 24-year-old man is seen in the ophthalmology outpatient department after referral by his general practitioner for recurrent attacks of uncomfortable red eyes. On closer questioning he describes a prodromal history of pain and morning stiffness to his lower back. On inspection of the affected eye injection is most pronounced around the iris, and his pupil is irregular in outline.

34 THEME: ACUTE LOSS OF VISION

A Acute closed-angle glaucoma
B Blunt traumatic loss of vision
C Endophthalmitis
D Giant cell (temporal) arteritis
E Ischaemic optic neuropathy
F Migraine
G Occipital lobe ischaemia
H Occipital lobe trauma
I Optic nerve trauma
J Optic neuritis
K Orbital cellulitis
L Penetrating traumatic loss of vision
M Raised intracranial pressure
N Retinal artery occlusion
O Retinal detachment
P Vitreous haemorrhage

The following patients all present complaining of acute visual loss. For each, please select the most appropriate diagnosis from the above list. The items may be used once, more than once, or not at all.

☐ **1** A 65-year-old man presents to the emergency eye department complaining of a sudden loss of vision in his right eye. On direct questioning you are able to elicit a history of right-sided scalp tenderness and recent malaise. Fundoscopy reveals haemorrhages on the disc and disc margin on the right, with cotton wool spots around the disc. His erythrocyte sedimentation rate is 118.

☐ **2** A 70-year-old woman attends her general practitioner's surgery with a history of a 'curtain' coming down rapidly in her left eye. She had a prior history of flashing lights and 'spots' floating in her vision. She has recently had surgery for a left-sided cataract.

☐ **3** A 60-year-old woman presents to The Emergency Department with a recurrent history of fleeting loss of vision in her left eye, often lasting up to 10 min. She tells you that she has just had another episode an hour earlier. On fundoscopy the acutely affected retina is swollen and white, and the fovea appears very red. You also notice that she has a bruit over her left carotid artery and the carotid pulse appears slightly diminished.

Principles of oncology

35 THEME: CHEMOTHERAPEUTIC AGENTS

A Bleomycin
B Chlorambucil
C Cisplatin
D Cyclophosphamide
E Docetaxel
F Doxorubicin
G Etoposide
H 5-Fluorouracil
I Flutamide
J Goserelin acetate
K Methotrexate
L Mitozantrone
M Oxaliplatin
N Tamoxifen
O Vincristine

The following are descriptions of chemotherapeutic agents used in surgical oncology. Please select the most appropriate agent from the above list. The items may be used once, more than once, or not at all.

☐ **1** A cytotoxic alkylating agent used to synergistically down-size liver metastases secondary to colorectal carcinoma.

☐ **2** The most widely used alkylating agent used in combination regimens for adjuvant chemotherapeutic treatment of node-positive, early-stage breast cancer.

☐ **3** A luteinising hormone-releasing hormone agonist used in T_{1-2} N_0 M_0 prostate cancer

☐ **4** The basis of nearly all regimens of adjuvant and palliative treatment of colorectal cancer.

36 THEME: CAUSES OF PAIN IN PALLIATIVE CARE

A Bone infiltration
B Candidiasis
C Capsular stretching
D Cranial neuralgia
E Deafferentation
F Lymphoedema
G Metastatic bone pain
H Muscular spasm
I Myofascial pain
J Nerve infiltration
K Peripheral nerve compression
L Peripheral polyneuropathy
M Soft tissue infiltration
N Spinal cord compression
O Ulceration
P Visceral infiltration

The following are descriptions of common causes of pain in palliative-care patients. Please select the most appropriate diagnosis from the above list. The items may be used once, more than once, or not at all.

☐ **1** A 57-year-old woman with advanced colorectal carcinoma complains of severe right-sided upper abdominal pain. On examination, although haemodynamically stable, she is exquisitely tender in the right upper quadrant.

☐ **2** A 72-year-old with advanced prostate carcinoma presents with severe lower back pain associated with sudden onset of weakness of the legs. On examination he has weakness and loss of sensation in both lower limbs; he has a palpably distended bladder; and rectal examination reveals a loaded rectum, yet lax anal sphincter tone.

☐ **3** A 60-year-old woman with left-sided buttock sarcoma complains of recent onset of worsening left-buttock pain, 'burning' in nature, extending down the back of the left leg to the ankle. On examination, there is decreased sensation at the back of the affected thigh and throughout the calf, inability to dorsiflex the left great toe, and a loss of the ankle reflex. An urgent spinal magnetic resonance imaging scan is unremarkable.

37 THEME: CANCER STAGING

A	Breslow staging	G	Gleason 8
B	Clark staging	H	Manchester staging
C	Dukes A	I	T_2, N_1, M_0
D	Dukes B	J	T_3, N_1, M_0
E	Gleason 3	K	T_3, N_2, M_0
F	Gleason 6	L	T_4, N_1, M_0

The above are all examples of cancer staging or a degree of staging. Please choose the most appropriate stage or staging system for the following descriptions of tumours. Each item may be used once, more than once, or not at all.

☐ **1** A pathological staging system, used in the assessment of malignant melanoma, based on measurement of depth of dermal tumour invasion.

☐ **2** A rectal adenocarcinoma that has penetrated through muscularis propria into peri-rectal fat. Seven of 12 nodes are histologically positive but there is no evidence of metastasis.

☐ **3** A splenic flexure adenocarcinoma that invades, but does not penetrate through, the muscularis propria. Histology rules out lymph node involvement and imaging techniques exclude metastases.

☐ **4** A moderately differentiated prostate cancer on histological assessment.

38 THEME: CANCER GENETICS

A *APC* gene
B Familial adenomatous polyposis
C Hereditary non-polyposis colorectal cancer
D Juvenile polyposis
E *K-RAS* gene
F Microsatellite instability
G Peutz–Jeghers syndrome
H *P53* gene
I Ulcerative colitis

The following are descriptions that refer to colorectal cancer genetics. Please select the most appropriate term from the list. The items may be used once, more than once, or not at all.

☐ **1** A condition accounting for approximately 3% of all cases of colorectal cancer, in which 40–80% of cases are caused by germ-line mutations in the mismatch repair genes *MLH1* and *MSH2*.

☐ **2** A hereditary autosomal dominant condition associated with multiple upper and lower gastrointestinal hamartomatous lesions and small bowel, pancreatic and colorectal cancer.

☐ **3** The most frequently observed activated oncogene in colorectal adenomas and carcinomas.

39 THEME: COMMON CARCINOGENS

A Arsenic
B Asbestos
C *Aspergillus flavus*
D Benzol/ benzene
E β-Naphthylamine
F Cyclophosphamide
G Diethyl stilboestrol
H Epstein–Barr virus
I Hardwood sawdust
J Hepatitis B virus
K Human immunodeficiency virus
L Human papillomavirus
M Human T-cell leukaemia virus type 1
N Nickel
O Nitrates/nitrites
P Nitrosamines/nitrosamides
Q Schistosomiasis
R Ultraviolet light
S Vinyl chloride monomer

The following scenarios describe patients who have had exposure to a carcinogen and subsequently developed a carcinoma. From the above list, choose the most appropriate carcinogen. Each item may be used once, more than once, or not at all.

☐ **1** A 70-year-old man presents with haematuria. Cystoscopy demonstrates a transitional cell carcinoma of the bladder. He had been in the paint industry all his working life.

☐ **2** A 47-year-old African immigrant presents with hepatomegaly. Imaging reveals a large solitary hepatic lesion. He tells you that he was a crop farmer growing cereal.

☐ **3** A 55-year-old man who stayed frequently in Egypt complains of haematuria. He also has suffered in the past with recurrent renal and bladder stones.

☐ **4** A 30-year-old woman presents with vaginal bleeding. A recent cervical smear shows high-grade cervical dysplasia.

SURGICAL SPECIALTIES

Cardiothoracic surgery

40 THEME: THORACIC TRAUMA

A Aortic disruption
B Cardiac tamponade
C Diaphragmatic rupture
D Flail chest
E Haemothorax
F Massive haemothorax
G Myocardial contusion
H Oesophageal rupture
I Open pneumothorax
J Pulmonary contusion
K Simple pneumothorax
L Tension pneumothorax
M Tracheobronchial disruption
N Traumatic asphyxia

The following patients have all had thoracic injuries. Please select the most appropriate diagnosis from the above list. The items may be used once, more than once, or not at all.

☐ **1** A 26-year-old soldier is hit by shrapnel, resulting in a large defect to the left side of his chest. He is brought to Casualty, the paramedics having securely occluded the defect on all sides with a sterile dressing. On examination he is severely dyspnoeic, tachycardic and hypotensive. His trachea is displaced to the right. Percussion reveals the left side of the chest to be hyper-resonant, with decreased air entry on auscultation.

☐ **2** A 65-year-old lady is brought to The Emergency Department having been involved in a road traffic accident; it was a head-on collision in which she was the driver. Her signs are initially stable, and examination only reveals bruising over and to the left of the sternum. A chest X-ray is normal. A few hours later she develops an irregular tachycardia confirmed by electrocardiogram to be atrial fibrillation.

☐ **3** A 50-year-old builder presents to The Emergency Department having been hit by falling scaffolding. He did not initially attend The Emergency Department; however, over the past few hours he has become increasingly dyspnoeic. On examination he has a respiratory rate of 30 breaths/min and a SaO_2 of 89%. He has equal air entry bilaterally and normal percussion. Chest X-ray reveals fractures of ribs 2 to 6 on the left side.

41 THEME: CHEST TRAUMA MANAGEMENT

A Arteriography
B Bilateral thoracostomy
C Computed tomography of thorax
D Emergency thoracotomy
E Immediate needle decompression
F Insertion of chest drain
G Intravenous access fluid resuscitation
H Intubation and ventilation
I Pericardiocentesis
J Resuscitation (emergency room) thoracotomy
K Transoesophageal echocardiography

The following patients have all had thoracic injuries. Please select the most appropriate management option from the above list. The items may be used once, more than once, or not at all.

☐ **1** A 27-year-old man is brought to The Emergency Department following a stab wound to the left side of the chest. On examination his respiratory rate is 24 breaths/min, pulse rate is 115/min, and blood pressure is 90/50 mmHg. There is a dull percussion note and decreased air entry on the affected side.

☐ **2** An 18-year-old woman is brought to The Emergency Department after being hit by a car travelling at approximately 50 miles/h. She has a suspected fractured pelvis and a Glasgow Coma Score of 13/15. On arrival, she has a respiratory rate of 36 breaths/min; pulse rate of 120/min and blood pressure is 90/60 mmHg. Examination reveals engorged neck veins, and a hyper-resonant percussion note on the left side of the chest. The background noise in the department renders auscultation of either breath or heart sounds difficult to assess.

☐ **3** A 65-year-old man is the driver in a high-speed road traffic accident. He is brought to The Emergency Department complaining of severe chest pain and difficulty breathing. Examination reveals a shallow respiratory rate of 34 breaths/min and a SaO_2 of 92% on 60% oxygen. He has contusions to both sides of the chest and there is reduced air entry bilaterally. Palpation of the chest wall reveals crepitus and asymmetrical movement of the right chest wall.

☐ **4** A 52-year-old window cleaner falls five storeys. He is brought to The Emergency Department with suspected bilateral hip dislocation and calcaneal fractures. He seems stable from a cardiorespiratory perspective. A chest X-ray taken as part of the routine trauma series reveals a widened mediastinum.

☐ **5** A 20-year-old is brought to The Emergency Department by paramedics having been stabbed to the left of the chest. He is intubated and ventilated and has been persistently hypotensive since scene. On transfer to the resuscitation bay he has a cardiac arrest.

42 THEME: LUNG CANCER: COMPLICATIONS

A Bony metastasis
B Cerebellar ataxia
C Clubbing
D Ectopic adrenocorticotropic hormone secretion
E Ectopic antidiuretic hormone secretion
F Ectopic parathyroid hormone secretion
G Intestinal pseudo-obstruction
H Isaac's syndrome
I Horner's syndrome
J Hypertrophic pulmonary osteoarthropathy
K Lambert–Eaton myasthenic syndrome
L Pancoast's syndrome
M Peripheral neuropathy
N Superior vena caval obstruction

The following patients all have lung cancer. Please select the most appropriate cause for the clinical findings in each case from the above list. The items may be used once, more than once, or not at all.

☐ **1** A 47-year-old smoker with a chronic cough attends his general practitioner with a history of severe pain in his left shoulder and radiating down his left arm. There is some weakness in the intrinsic muscles of the left hand. Sputum cytology reveals malignant keratinised cells.

☐ **2** A 75-year-old lady is brought in by ambulance after being found collapsed by neighbours. On examination she is drowsy and becomes agitated when attempts are made to rouse her. Routine observations show that her blood pressure is 170/95 mmHg and heart rate is 72 bpm. Her biochemistry results come back as urea & electrolytes: Na^+ 116 mmol/litre, K^+ 3.0 mmol/litre, urea 6.5 mmol/litre, creatinine 92 μmol/litre; plasma osmolality: 251 mosmol/kg.

☐ **3** A 67-year-old man with lung cancer is seen by the palliative-care team after complaining of severe fatigue and weakness. He is now unable to stand from sitting, has problems chewing and gets occasional double vision. Examination shows normal power in the hands and feet, but weakness of the girdle muscles and an oculomotor nerve palsy on the right with ptosis. The doctor is surprised that the weakness improves after repeated demonstrations to colleagues.

General surgery

43 THEME: COMMON ABDOMINAL OPERATIONS

A Abdomino-perineal excision of rectum
B Anterior resection of rectum
C Completion colectomy
D Hartmann's procedure
E Laparoscopic cholecystectomy
F Loop colostomy
G Left hemicolectomy
H On-table lavage, primary resection and anastomosis
I Restorative proctocolectomy
J Right hemicolectomy
K Stricturoplasty
L Total mesorectal excision

The following patients are all to undergo surgery. Please select the most appropriate operation from the above list. The items may be used once, more than once, or not at all.

☐ **1** You have seen a 74-year-old man in The Emergency Department. He gives a 3-day history of localised lower abdominal pain, which has become generalised over the past 24 h. He is known to suffer with ischaemic heart disease and sigmoid diverticulosis. On examination he is dehydrated, tachycardic (pulse 120/min), pale, sweating and pyrexial (38 °C). Abdominal examination reveals the presence of diffuse abdominal tenderness, guarding and rigidity. The results of investigations performed so far have demonstrated a raised white cell count of 22.5×10^9/litre, acidosis on arterial blood gases and pneumoperitoneum on erect chest X-ray.

☐ **2** A 23-year-old man with long-standing Crohn's disease is seen in the combined colitis clinic. He gives you a long history from adolescence of recurrent episodes of colicky abdominal pain and vomiting. A recent colonoscopy has not demonstrated any significant colonic pathology and, in addition, he has had a barium meal and follow-through, which has been reported as demonstrating significant terminal ileal stricturing. He continues to be symptomatic and is now keen on having surgery.

☐ **3** A 64-year-old woman has been seen in the rectal bleed clinic and a diagnosis of a low rectal cancer (7 cm from the anal verge) has been made. A magnetic resonance imaging scan demonstrates a resectable lesion.

44 THEME: HERNIAS (TYPES AND TAXONOMY)

A Femoral hernia
B Gluteal hernia
C Incarcerated hernia
D Incisional hernia
E Internal hernia
F Littre's hernia
G Lumbar hernia
H Maydl's hernia
I Obstructed hernia
J Obturator hernia
K Richter's hernia
L Spigelian hernia
M Strangulated hernia

The following patients all have hernias. From the list above, select the most appropriate diagnosis, according to the clinical and/or anatomical information provided. The items may be used once, more than once, or not at all.

☐ **1** A 48-year-old gentleman presents with a 36-h history of vomiting, central abdominal pain and distension. On examination, he is unwell, febrile, dehydrated and tachycardic. Abdominal examination reveals a distended abdomen with 'tinkling' bowel sounds, and a very large right inguino-scrotal hernia that is irreducible, erythematous and tender. At operation, a W-loop of small bowel lies in the hernial sac.

☐ **2** A 49-year-old woman is admitted with acute small bowel obstruction. She reports a 2-day history of severe pain radiating down the inner aspect of the right thigh to her knee. Consequently, you meticulously examine the hernial orifices in the groin, but **no** hernia is evident. Ultimately, she requires a laparotomy, as her obstruction fails to resolve with conservative management. Only then does the cause of her obstruction become apparent.

☐ **3** A 65-year-old gentleman attends the outpatients department with a long history of an intermittent swelling in the right groin that is now persistent. The swelling is irreducible but is non-tender, and lies above and medial to the pubic tubercle. He denies any gastro-intestinal disturbance.

45 THEME: MANAGEMENT OF GROIN HERNIAS

A Bassini repair
B Herniogram
C Herniotomy
D Laparoscopic intraperitoneal repair
E Lichtenstein repair
F Low crural (Lockwood) approach
G High crural (Lothiessan) approach
H McEvedie's approach (or modification)
I Shouldice procedure
J Totally extraperitoneal prosthetic repair (TEPP)
K Transabdominal preperitoneal prosthetic repair (TAPP)
L Truss
M Ultrasound scan

The following patients have all presented with groin hernias. Select the most appropriate management option. Each option may be used once, more than once, or not at all.

☐ **1** An 80-year-old woman is admitted to hospital with a 20-h history of abdominal distension, pain and vomiting. On examination, there is a small tender lump lying below and lateral to the pubic tubercle with overlying erythema. The patient has been fully resuscitated.

☐ **2** A 56-year-old man presents at outpatients with a small reducible inguinal hernia. You are a trainee of the Royal College of Surgeons of England and must perform the repair.

☐ **3** A 32-year-old man presents to outpatients from the general practitioner complaining of a small lump in the groin that comes and goes and causes pain when present. On examination you find no evidence of hernia.

☐ **4** A 2-year-old boy is brought in with a right groin lump. This proves reducible with sedation, analgesia and cold packs. It is planned for him to return for day-case surgery in 48 h.

46 THEME: GROIN LUMPS

A Ectopic testis
B Femoral artery aneurysm
C Femoral hernia
D Hydrocoele of the spermatic cord
E Inguinal hernia
F Inguinal lymphadenopathy
G Lipoma
H Pseudo-aneurysm
I Psoas abscess
J Psoas bursa
K Saphena varix
L Sarcoma

The following patients all present with a lump in the groin. For each scenario please select the most appropriate diagnosis from the above list. The items may be used once, more than once, or not at all.

☐ **1** A 36-year-old Asian immigrant presents to The Emergency Department with a tender, fluctuant mass in his left femoral triangle. He gives a history of night sweats, weight loss and a painful left hip.

☐ **2** A 68-year-old man attends Casualty suffering from drowsiness and confusion. His wife reports a 12-h history of vomiting and abdominal pain. On examination he is clearly dehydrated, his abdomen is distended and he has high-pitched bowel sounds. More detailed assessment reveals a small painful swelling in his right groin crease.

☐ **3** A 62-year-old claudicant returns to the ward from the vascular assessment laboratory, following an angiogram of his lower limbs. The nurse is concerned about a swelling in his left groin. On closer examination you note a firm mass with a transmissible pulse.

47 THEME: RIGHT ILIAC FOSSA MASS

A	Actinomycosis	H	Ovarian carcinoma
B	Appendix abscess	I	Ovarian cyst
C	Appendix mass	J	Pelvic kidney
D	Caecal carcinoma	K	Psoas abscess
E	Crohn's disease	L	Ruptured epigastric artery
F	Iliac artery aneurysm	M	Tuberculous ileitis
G	Iliac lymphadenopathy	N	Tumour in undescended testis

The following are descriptions of patients with a right iliac fossa mass. Please select the most appropriate diagnosis from the list. The items may be used once, more than once, or not at all.

☐ **1** An 18-year-old man presents to The Emergency Department with a 7-day history of colicky right iliac fossa pain associated with a persistent fever and anorexia. On examination, the patient has a temperature of 37.8 °C, pulse rate 98/min, and there is a tender indistinct mass in the right iliac fossa.

☐ **2** A 31-year-old woman is referred to the outpatient clinic with a 1-year history of recurrent episodes of pain in the right iliac fossa, associated with an increased frequency of passing loose stool. On further questioning, she admits to a weight loss of 1 stone over the same time period. On examination there is a tender mass in the right iliac fossa.

☐ **3** A 67-year-old woman presents to clinic with anaemia, unexplained weight loss and non-specific lower abdominal pain. On examination there is a distinct hard mobile mass.

48 THEME: THE ACUTE ABDOMEN: INVESTIGATION AND MANAGEMENT

A Appendicectomy
B Computed tomography scan
C Diagnostic laparoscopy
D Laparoscopic appendicectomy
E Laparotomy
F Regular clinical review
G Ultrasound scan

The following scenarios describe patients with various causes of acute abdominal pain. Assuming that they have undergone resuscitation and basic investigation, choose from the list above the most appropriate next step in management. Each item may be used once, more than once, or not at all.

☐ **1** A 70-year-old, hypertensive smoker with a 3-h history of sudden onset of worsening lower back pain and bilateral lower limb paralysis.

☐ **2** An 80-year-old woman presents with a 24-h history of absolute constipation associated with lower abdominal pain. On examination, she is grossly distended with localised peritonism in the right iliac fossa. The plain film demonstrates large bowel obstruction.

☐ **3** A 26-year-old woman presents with a 14-h history of right iliac fossa pain, associated with nausea and vomiting. On examination there is tenderness and guarding in the right iliac fossa. She reports, however, that her pain is similar to an episode she had 1 year ago when she torted an ovarian cyst and required surgery.

☐ **4** A 38-year-old man with a previous history of alcoholic pancreatitis presents with a 12-h history of increasingly severe epigastric pain and vomiting. On examination, he is dehydrated, tachycardic and has widespread abdominal peritonism. White cell count 16.2×10^9/litre, amylase 340. No free gas found on erect chest X-ray.

49 THEME: THE ACUTE ABDOMEN

A Acute cholecystitis
B Acute pancreatitis
C Appendicitis
D Biliary colic
E Diverticulitis
F Gastroduodenitis
G Large bowel obstruction
H Leaking abdominal aortic aneurysm
I Meckel's diverticulum
J Mesenteric infarction
K Ovarian cyst torsion
L Perforated duodenal ulcer
M Small bowel obstruction
N Ureteric colic

The following scenarios describe patients presenting with acute abdominal pain. From the above list, choose the most likely cause. Each item may be used once, more than once, or not all.

☐ **1** A 78-year-old woman presents with a 4-h history of very severe constant central abdominal pain. She looks very unwell and is in distress despite diamorphine. Examination reveals slight abdominal distension with some central tenderness but no peritonism. She is afebrile, blood pressure 140/90 mmHg, pulse 95/min irregularly irregular and respiratory rate 30 breaths/min. Blood gases pH 7.1, $p_A(O_2)$ 11 kPa, $p_A(CO_2)$ 4.6 kPa, HCO_3^- 18 mmol/litre, base excess −6.

☐ **2** A 75-year-old man presents with a 12-h history of worsening left iliac fossa pain associated with an exacerbation of his usual constipation. Assessment reveals a temperature of 38.2 °C and tenderness and guarding in the left iliac fossa. White cell count 18.2 × 10^9/litre, haemoglobin 14.1 g/dl, C-reactive protein 150.

☐ **3** A 39-year-old man presents with sudden-onset, right-sided colicky abdominal pain that he describes as 'the worst he's had in his life'. Abdominal examination is unremarkable.

50 THEME: EPIGASTRIC PAIN/DYSPEPSIA: MANAGEMENT

- A Barium swallow
- B Coeliac axis angiography
- C Computed tomography scan – chest/abdomen
- D Emergency laparotomy
- E Erect chest X-ray
- F *Helicobacter pylori* eradication therapy
- G Injection sclerotherapy
- H Nissen's fundoplication
- I Oesophageal manometry
- J Prokinetic drug
- K Proton pump inhibitor
- L Serum gastrin
- M Thermal coagulation

The following are all descriptions of endoscopic findings in patients who are being investigated for oesophageal/gastroduodenal disorders. Please select the next most appropriate course of action from the list above. This may be an investigation or a form of treatment. The items may be used once, more than once, or not at all.

☐ **1** A 48-year-old woman is under investigation for epigastric pain. An upper gastrointestinal endoscopy has been performed, which demonstrated the presence of friable lower oesophageal mucosa and linear ulceration.

☐ **2** A 65-year-old man has been brought into the resuscitation room with repeated bouts of haematemesis. An upper gastrointestinal endoscopy is performed as an emergency, which demonstrates a large volume of blood in the stomach and duodenum. Repeated efforts to control the rate of bleeding endoscopically have failed.

☐ **3** A 72-year-old woman is seen with a history of weight loss and progressive dysphagia. At endoscopy a friable, polypoid fungating growth is noted in the region of the gastro-oesophageal junction from which biopsies have been taken.

☐ **4** A 35-year-old diabetic has been referred with a history of vomiting, abdominal bloating and early satiety. At endoscopy a dilated stomach full of stale food is noted. However, no obstructing lesion or stricture is detected and the endoscope passes easily into the duodenum.

51 THEME: RIGHT ILIAC FOSSA PAIN (COMMON CAUSES)

A Acute appendicitis
B Caecal carcinoma
C Crohn's disease
D Diverticulitis
E Gastroenteritis
F Irritable bowel syndrome
G Mesenteric adenitis
H Non-specific abdominal pain
I Pelvic inflammatory disease
J Ruptured ectopic pregnancy
K Torsion ovarian cyst
L Ureteric colic
M Urinary tract infection

The following are descriptions of patients with common causes of right iliac fossa pain. Please select the most appropriate diagnosis from the list. The items may be used once, more than once, or not at all.

☐ **1** A 22-year-old man is seen in The Emergency Department with a 2-day history of right iliac fossa pain, anorexia, vomiting and diarrhoea. On examination the patient is flushed and tachycardic (pulse 100/min). Abdominal examination demonstrates the presence of tenderness and guarding in the right iliac fossa with no masses palpable.

☐ **2** A 38-year-old woman is seen in the outpatients department with a 1-year history of right-sided abdominal pain that is often relieved following defaecation. On direct questioning she describes a change in her bowel habit with alternating diarrhoea and constipation along with recurrent abdominal distension. She has no loss in weight, or rectal bleeding. On examination she appears well and her abdomen is soft with no obvious distension. Blood tests and a supine abdominal radiograph are all normal.

☐ **3** A 26-year-old woman is seen in The Emergency Department with a history of increasingly severe right iliac fossa pain, which made her faint. In addition, she complains of feeling weak, thirsty and has developed pain in her right shoulder. She describes no gynaecological symptoms. On examination she is pale, clammy and has a sinus tachycardia of 115 bpm. Examination of her abdomen reveals diffuse tenderness, guarding and distension across her lower abdomen.

☐ **4** A 23-year-old woman presents to The Emergency Department with a history of sudden onset severe right iliac fossa pain 4 hours ago. She has tenderness and guarding localised to the right iliac fossa and suprapubic region.

52 THEME: RIGHT ILIAC FOSSA PAIN (RARE CAUSES)

A Diverticulitis
B Fractured NOF
C Ileocaecal tuberculosis
D Leaking iliac aneurysm
E Lymphoma
F Meckel's diverticulitis
G Psoas abscess
H Rectus sheath haematoma
I Ruptured corpus luteum cyst
J Strangulated spigelian hernia
K Tabes dorsalis
L Torsion of an undescended testis

The following are descriptions of patients with rare causes of right iliac fossa pain. Please select the most appropriate diagnosis from the list. The items may be used once, more than once, or not at all.

☐ **1** A 23-year-old amateur footballer presents with a 12-h history of right iliac fossa pain. The pain started while running and has become increasingly severe since. There is no history of fever or vomiting. On examination he is in obvious discomfort and has a very tender mass palpable low in the right iliac fossa.

☐ **2** A 29-year-old Indian man presents with a 1-month history of pain in his right iliac fossa. On direct questioning he says he has felt unwell over the past 6 months with a history of malaise, anorexia and pain in his lumbar spine and right groin. On examination he is thin and appears malnourished. Abdominal examination reveals the presence of vague tenderness in the right iliac fossa and loin, in addition to a fluctuant lump in his groin on the same side.

53 THEME: CHRONIC NON-MALIGNANT PELVIC PAIN IN WOMEN

A Benign ovarian tumour
B Complications of uterine leiomyomata
C Chronic constipation
D Degenerative changes of the lumbar spine
E Diverticular disease
F Endometriosis
G Inflammatory bowel disease
H Irritable bowel syndrome
I Painful bladder syndrome
J Pelvic adhesions
K Pelvic congestion syndrome
L Pelvic inflammatory disease
M Recurrent cystitis
N Urolithiasis
O Utero-vaginal prolapse

The following female patients present with chronic non-malignant pelvic pain. From the list above, select the most likely diagnosis. The items may be used once, more than once, or not at all.

☐ **1** A 58-year-old librarian attends outpatients with a 12-month history of pelvic pain. She describes the pain as 'dragging' in nature, and reports that it is worse towards the 'end of her working day'. She also complains of difficulty voiding, and a sensation of incomplete emptying following defaecation. She had four children before undergoing a premature menopause at the age of 40 years. She takes no regular medication.

☐ **2** A 24-year-old woman presents with a chronic history of pelvic pain following the birth of her first child. She has no relevant lower gastrointestinal, urological, or gynaecological symptoms. Abdominal examination of the abdomen reveals a non-tender mass in the left iliac fossa. There is no clinical evidence of ascites or organomegaly.

☐ **3** A 42-year-old woman is referred by her general practitioner (GP) with a 3-year history of disabling supra-pubic pain that has resulted in repeated absence from work. Her GP states that her urinalysis and repeated urine cultures have all been negative, and that she has no relevant gynaecological history of note. The GP suspects that her pain is the result of 'bowel pathology', and asks for your assessment. On direct questioning, the patient describes urinary frequency and urgency. She has no gastrointestinal symptoms. Examination is unremarkable.

☐ **4** A 65-year-old woman presents with a long history of constipation and abdominal bloating. More recently, she has been troubled with severe intermittent left iliac fossa pain. Looking through her notes, you notice a recent admission with 'brisk bleeding per rectum'. She tells you that she is awaiting a colonoscopy. She is post-menopausal and has no urinary symptoms. Current medication includes Fybogel and hormone replacement therapy.

54 THEME: THE ABDOMINAL MASS

A Abdominal aortic aneurysm
B Appendix mass
C Carcinoma of the caecum
D Carcinoma of the head of the pancreas
E Carcinoma of the sigmoid colon
F Carcinoma of the stomach
G Crohn's mass
H Diverticular mass
I Empyema of the gallbladder
J Hepatomegaly
K Mesenteric cyst
L Mucocoele of the gallbladder
M Pancreatic pseudocyst
N Renal cell carcinoma
O Splenomegaly

The following patients have all presented with a palpable abdominal mass. Please select the most appropriate diagnosis from the above list. The items may be used once, more than once, or not at all.

☐ **1** A 57-year-old woman presents with a 6-month history of a dull ache in the right iliac fossa associated with anorexia and lethargy. The pain has become acute over the past week with episodes of peri-umbilical colic and abdominal distension, which is relieved on vomiting. On examination the patient is pale and dehydrated. Abdominal examination reveals the presence of generalised abdominal distension and a firm, irregular mass in the right iliac fossa.

☐ **2** A 56-year-old woman presents with a 2-week history of increasing jaundice and pruritis. Direct questioning reveals that over the past few months she has had some vague epigastric pain, radiating to the back. On examination a smooth hemi-ovoid mass is palpable in the right upper quadrant, which moves with respiration. It is dull to percussion.

☐ **3** An 18-year-old woman presents with a history of a painless, central abdominal swelling. She is concerned, as this has gradually increased in size without causing any symptoms. On examination she is anxious but otherwise appears well. Abdominal examination reveals a fluctuant, spherical mass near the umbilicus. Of note, the mass is mobile, frequently 'slipping' towards the left iliac fossa during palpation.

55 THEME: HEPATOMEGALY

A	Amyloid disease	H	Hydatid disease
B	Biliary tract obstruction	I	Infective hepatitis
C	Cardiac failure	J	Leukaemia
D	Cirrhosis	K	Liver abscess
E	Haemochromatosis	L	Lymphoma
F	Hepatocellular carcinoma	M	Metastatic carcinoma
G	Hepatic vein obstruction (Budd–Chiari syndrome)	N	Polycystic disease
		O	Riedel's lobe

The above are all causes of discrete or diffuse liver enlargement. For the scenarios below please select the most appropriate diagnosis from the list. The items may be used once, more than once, or not at all.

☐ **1** A well 35-year-old woman is referred to you in the surgical outpatients by her concerned general practitioner (GP). In his letter he documents an enlarged liver. On examination, you notice a smooth mass extending from the costal margin towards the right iliac fossa. Liver function tests requested by her GP are normal.

☐ **2** A 58-year-old African man presents to The Emergency Department complaining of a 3-week history of 'gnawing' right upper quadrant pain, weight loss and abdominal distension. His history reveals that he had a blood transfusion in his home country after his involvement in a severe road traffic accident 10 years previously. Examination reveals jaundice, a nodular and enlarged liver, and the presence of shifting dullness.

56 THEME: CONDITIONS THAT MAY REQUIRE SPLENECTOMY

A Autoimmune haemolytic anaemia
B Chronic myeloid leukaemia
C Congenital spherocytosis
D Felty's syndrome
E Gaucher's disease
F Hodgkin's lymphoma
G Idiopathic thrombocytic purpura
H Myelofibrosis
I Sickle cell disease
J Splenic abscess
K Thalassaemia
L Trauma
M Tropical splenomegaly

The following are descriptions of patients with splenomegaly. Please select the most appropriate diagnosis from the list. The items may be used once, more than once, or not at all.

☐ **1** A 13-year-old boy is referred with intermittent colicky right upper quadrant pain. Examination reveals clinical anaemia, jaundice and splenomegaly. Abdominal ultrasound reveals a moderately enlarged spleen and multiple, small gallstone calculi.

☐ **2** A 50-year-old man, with a 3-year history of fatigue, weight loss and anorexia, is referred for recent onset of a dragging sensation in the upper abdomen. Examination reveals generalised lymphadenopathy and massive splenomegaly.

☐ **3** A 26-year-old woman, with a history of intravenous drug abuse, presents with severe upper left abdominal pain, fever and rigors. On examination she is tachycardic and pyrexial with a mildly enlarged tender spleen.

57 THEME: COMPLICATIONS OF SPLENECTOMY

A Basal atelectasis
B Deep vein thrombosis
C Gastric perforation
D Gastric stasis
E Lower lobe pneumonia
F Overwhelming post-splenectomy sepsis
G Pancreatic fistula
H Pancreatic pseudocyst
I Portal vein thrombosis
J Pulmonary embolus
K Splenosis
L Subphrenic abscess

The following are descriptions of patients with post-splenectomy complications. Please select the most appropriate diagnosis from the list. The items may be used once, more than once, or not at all.

☐ **1** A 13-year-old boy presents to The Emergency Department with a severe headache and vomiting; for the past 2 to 3 days he has been off school for presumed influenza. On examination he is flushed and has a temperature of 39 °C. There are no specific findings; however, on further questioning his parents state that he had an emergency splenectomy following a road traffic accident 1 year ago.

☐ **2** A 42-year-old woman complains of left-sided chest and abdominal pain, worse on inspiration, 7 days post-splenectomy. Examination reveals a temperature of 38.6 °C, decreased air entry at the left lung base, dullness to percussion and left upper quadrant tenderness.

58 THEME: INTESTINAL OBSTRUCTION

A Adhesions
B Bezoar
C Colonic carcinoma
D Crohn's disease
E Colonic pseudo-obstruction
F Diverticular disease
G Extra-luminal neoplastic compression
H Gallstone ileus
I Hernia
J Intussusception
K Intestinal pseudo-obstruction
L Small bowel tumour
M Volvulus

The following scenarios describe patients with signs of obstruction. From the above list choose the most likely cause. Each item may be used once, more than once, or not at all.

☐ **1** A 75-year-old woman presents with an 8-h history of vomiting and colicky central abdominal pain. Her abdomen appears mildly distended and although she is uncomfortable, there is no obvious tenderness. A plain abdominal radiograph demonstrates pneumobilia.

☐ **2** An 88-year-old man is admitted from a nursing home with confusion, lower abdominal pain and gross distension. A plain abdominal radiograph demonstrates the 'coffee-bean sign'.

☐ **3** A 30-year-old man presents with a several month history of right-sided abdominal pain and some diarrhoea and weight loss. Subsequent radiological investigations demonstrate the 'string sign of Kantor'.

☐ **4** A 78-year-old man with known small cell carcinoma of the lung attends with abdominal pain, distension and vomiting. The abdomen is soft and non-tender with no masses. He has had no previous abdominal surgery and there is no hernia.

59 THEME: LARGE BOWEL OBSTRUCTION

A Caecal carcinoma
B Caecal volvulus
C Carcinoma
D Diverticular disease
E Faecal impaction
F Foreign body
G Intussusception
H Ischaemic stricture
I Pelvic metastases
J Pseudo-obstruction
K Sigmoid volvulus

The following patients have all presented with large bowel obstruction. Please select the most appropriate diagnosis from the above list. The items may be used once, more than once, or not at all.

☐ **1** A 67-year-old woman presents with a 4-day history of colicky, central abdominal pain and increasing distension. She gives a long history of a tendency towards constipation; however, on this occasion she has not opened her bowels for 2 weeks, nor has she passed any flatus. She describes episodes of left-sided abdominal pain over the preceding 6 years. Her weight and appetite are unchanged. On examination she is dehydrated and in obvious discomfort. Her abdomen is distended, tympanic to percussion and a vague mass is palpable in the left iliac fossa. An empty rectum is found on rectal examination.

☐ **2** A 42-year-old man undergoes a posterior L4–L5 spinal fixation. You are asked to review him on the second post-operative day. He has gross distension but a soft non-tender abdomen. He has not passed wind since the operation.

☐ **3** A 60-year-old man is seen in the resuscitation area of The Emergency Department. The nurse looking after him has moved him there because of his history of an abdominal aortic aneurysm repair 14 weeks earlier. He gives a 7-day history of lower abdominal pain associated with abdominal distension. He has not opened his bowels over the past 3 days, nor has he passed any flatus. This is unusual as he has had severe diarrhoea since his operation, which his general practitioner says is the result of an infection he 'picked up' while in hospital.

60 THEME: ABDOMINAL DISTENSION

A Ascites
B Constipation
C Gastric outflow obstruction
D Haemoperitoneum
E Large bowel obstruction
F Massive hepatomegaly
G Massive splenomegaly
H Obesity
I Ovarian cyst/tumour
J Paralytic ileus
K Pregnancy
L Pseudomyxoma peritonei
M Retroperitoneal sarcoma
N Small bowel obstruction
O Urinary bladder
P Uterine fibroids

The following patients have all presented with abdominal distension. Please select the most appropriate diagnosis from the above list. The items may be used once, more than once, or not at all.

☐ **1** A 53-year-old woman is referred by her general practitioner with a long history of increasing abdominal distension. In addition, she complains of increased frequency of micturition and worsening shortness of breath. On examination she is dyspnoeic at rest but otherwise comfortable. She has a large, palpable mass occupying her lower abdomen. The upper limit extends above the umbilicus. The lower limit is impalpable and, of note, the mass is resonant on percussion.

☐ **2** A 39-year-old man is seen in the outpatient department with a history of a left-sided abdominal swelling associated with pain in his left loin. He has lost his appetite and lost 22 kg (3 stones) in weight. Furthermore, he complains of constipation and has had episodes of colicky abdominal pain that resolve with the passage of loose stools. On examination he is thin with a grossly distended abdomen. A smooth, non-tender mass with vague margins is palpable. The mass can be balloted on the left side.

☐ **3** A 22-year-old final year medical student is seen in the occupational health department with a 2-week history of general malaise and headaches. Over the past two days she has been complaining of hot and cold sweats associated with rigors and vomiting. She has not felt right since returning from her elective in Papua New Guinea 2 months earlier. On examination she is thin and appears flushed. Her abdomen is distended. A firm, smooth mass, occupying the left half of her abdomen is found on palpation.

61 THEME: DYSPHAGIA

A Achalasia
B Bulbar palsy
C Chagas' disease
D CREST (calcinosis, Raynaud phenomenon, oesophageal motility disorders, sclerodactyly, telangiectasia)
E Diffuse oesophageal spasm
F Foreign bodies
G Gastro-oesophageal reflux disease
H Myasthenia gravis
I Oesophageal candidiasis
J Oesophageal carcinoma
K Paraoesophageal hernia
L Pharyngeal pouch (Zenker's diverticulum)
M Pharyngeal web
N Pseudobulbar palsy
O Scleroderma

The following patients have all presented with difficulty swallowing (dysphagia). Please select the most appropriate diagnosis from the above list. The items may be used once, more than once, or not at all.

☐ **1** A 40-year-old woman presents with a history of intermittent severe chest pains and dysphagia. Cardiac investigations are normal and the patient is eventually sent to a gastroenterologist for review. A gastroscopy is normal but subsequent oesophageal manometry reveals a pattern of contractions that occur simultaneously with episodes of chest pain.

☐ **2** A 37-year-old man presents with a 6-month history of progressive difficulty with speech and swallowing. On examination there is some weakness of facial muscles bilaterally with drooling. The tongue is flaccid and shows fasciculation, and the jaw jerk is absent. Eye movements are normal.

☐ **3** A 69-year-old Brazilian presents with a 3-month history of difficulty swallowing. He initially felt solids sticking at chest level but now has difficulty drinking. He has lost 8 kg in weight. Examination is unremarkable apart from his gaunt appearance.

62 THEME: VOMITING

A Drug-related
B Central neuronal causes
C Cholecystitis
D Enteritis
E Gastritis
F Metabolic/endocrine
G Obstruction
H Pancreatitis
I Peptic ulcer disease

The following patients have all presented with nausea and vomiting. Please select the most appropriate diagnosis from the above list. The items may be used once, more than once, or not at all.

☐ **1** A 23-year-old man attends The Emergency Department on a Sunday night with nausea, vomiting and epigastric pain. On examination, there is little to find other than mild epigastric tenderness. Investigations are normal.

☐ **2** A 56-year-old woman is 1-day post uncomplicated laparoscopic cholecystectomy. She is due to go home but has persistent nausea and vomiting.

63 THEME: INVESTIGATION AND MANAGEMENT OF GASTROINTESTINAL BLEEDING

A Angiography
B Barium meal
C Colectomy
D Colonoscopy
E Double contrast barium enema
F Emergency underun of bleeding ulcer
G Flexible sigmoidoscopy
H OGD and adrenaline injection
I OGD and banding
J OGD and sclerotherapy
K Partial gastrectomy
L Proctosigmoidoscopy
M Red cell radionucleotide scanning

The above are all methods of investigating or treating gastrointestinal bleeding. For the following scenarios please pick the most appropriate answer from the list. Each item may be used once, more than once, or not at all. In these scenarios it is taken for granted that all patients are appropriately resuscitated in the first instance.

☐ **1** A 57-year-old man presents with significant haematemesis and melaena. After resuscitation he undergoes upper gastrointestinal endoscopy. This highlights an actively bleeding duodenal ulcer with visible vessels at its base.

☐ **2** A 30-year-old man presents to The Emergency Department with a short history of bright red bleeding per rectum. On questioning he has a long history of noticing blood on the paper and occasionally in the toilet pan. He is otherwise well; Haemoglobin is 13.7 g/dl.

☐ **3** A 63-year-old woman presents with a history of melaena that is increasing in frequency. Her last few motions have also contained fresh dark red blood; haemoglobin 10.9 g/dl. An upper gastrointestinal endoscopy is normal and an unprepared colonoscopy cannot clearly identify a source of acute bleeding. Despite adequate fluid resuscitation she continues to exhibit signs of hypovolaemia and a repeat haemoglobin is 7.0 g/dl. A blood transfusion is commenced and although relatively stable, further intervention is clearly necessary.

64 THEME: HAEMATEMESIS

A Acute erosive gastritis
B Aortic enteric fistula
C Dieulafoy's syndrome (gastric arteriovenous malformation)
D Duodenal ulcer
E Gastric adenocarcinoma
F Gastric leiomyoma
G Gastric ulcer
H Mallory–Weiss tear
I Oesophageal carcinoma
J Oesophageal varices
K Oesophagitis
L Zollinger–Ellison syndrome

The above are all possible causes of haematemesis. From the following clinical scenarios please pick the most appropriate diagnosis from the list. Each item may be used once, more than once, or not at all.

☐ **1** A 40-year-old man presents to Casualty complaining of several episodes of coffee-ground vomiting. He has been taking ibuprofen for 4 weeks for shoulder pain related to an exercise-induced injury. He tells you that he has been regularly troubled by bouts of epigastric pain over the past year. This worsens in relation to stresses at work and is eased by eating. Full blood count: haemoglobin 11.8 g/dl, white cell count 7.4×10^9/litre, platelets 200×10^9/litre, mean corpuscular volume 84, INR 1.0.

☐ **2** A 67-year-old man is brought into The Emergency Department by his family. He is vomiting small amounts of fresh blood. His wife tells you that he has been complaining of a gnawing upper abdominal pain for nearly 2 months but has put it down to indigestion and stress at work. She is also worried about his weight loss and poor appetite (can only eat a little at a time). Full blood count: haemoglobin 9.4 g/dl, white cell count 6.0×10^9/litre, platelets 390×10^9/litre, mean corpuscular volume 68, INR 1.0.

☐ **3** An unkempt man is brought into majors by ambulance. He is vomiting copious amounts of fresh red blood. On examination, he is drowsy and you notice (after initial resuscitation is instituted) that he has clinical ascites. Full blood count: haemoglobin 7.4 g/dl, white cell count 12.0×10^9/litre, platelets 190×10^9/litre, mean corpuscular volume 102, INR 1.9.

65 THEME: INVESTIGATION AND MANAGEMENT OF GASTROINTESTINAL PERFORATION

A Cervical exploration and drainage
B Colonic resection and primary anastomosis
C Conservative treatment (antibiotics, total parenteral nutrition, nasogastric tube)
D Computed tomography scan +/− guided drainage
E Emergency gastrectomy
F Emergency thoracotomy
G Gastrograffin enema
H Gastrograffin swallow
I Hartmann's procedure
J Oesophageal resection
K Oesophageal stenting
L Omental patch repair
M Primary repair and drainage (oesophagus)
N Upper gastrointestinal endoscopy

The above are all methods of evaluating or managing gastrointestinal perforation. For each of the following clinical presentations please choose the most appropriate answer from the list. Each item may be used once, more than once, or not at all.

☐ **1** A previously fit 50-year-old man presents to The Emergency Department complaining of retrosternal pain radiating to his back, on a background of 24 h of dysphagia. He tells you that he underwent an upper gastrointestinal endoscopy for chronic dyspeptic symptoms 3 days earlier. Apparently the procedure had been difficult, requiring multiple attempts to intubate the oesophagus, before being abandoned. On examination he has mild crepitus in the soft tissues around his neck and auscultation reveals a positive Hamman's sign. His temperature is 38.3 °C, blood pressure 130/75 mmHg, pulse 105/min. Water-soluble contrast swallow shows a small localised leak in the region of the thoracic oesophagus.

☐ **2** A 64-year-old woman presents to Casualty with a 24-h history of progressive left iliac fossa pain. She has been conservatively treated for diverticulitis in the past (with prior barium enema confirming sigmoid disease). On examination, she has localised tenderness and guarding in the left iliac fossa. In addition, her temperature is 38.9 °C, blood pressure 105/60 mmHg, pulse 110/min.

66 THEME: JAUNDICE

A Acute viral hepatitis
B Alcoholic cirrhosis
C Ascending cholangitis
D Carcinoma of the gallbladder
E Cholangiocarcinoma
F Hepatocellular carcinoma
G Lymphoma
H Multiple hepatic metastases
I Pancreatic carcinoma
J Primary biliary cirrhosis
K Primary sclerosing cholangitis
L Stone in the common bile duct (CBD)

The following are descriptions of patients with jaundice. Please select the most appropriate diagnosis from the above list. The items may be used once, more than once, or not at all.

☐ **1** A 74-year-old woman is seen in The Emergency Department with a 4-week history of progressive jaundice and pruritis. On direct questioning, she has a 3-month history of anorexia and weight loss. On examination, she is cachectic, deeply icteric with evidence of weight loss. The gallbladder is palpable with no obvious hepatomegaly.

☐ **2** A 57-year-old man presents with a 5-week history of right upper quadrant pain, weight loss and increasing jaundice. He is a known hepatitis B carrier. On examination he is wasted and obviously jaundiced. Examination of his abdomen reveals a stony hard mass in the right upper quadrant that extends across his epigastrium.

☐ **3** A 49-year-old woman presents with recent onset of jaundice. On further questioning she has noticed bouts of pruritis and dark urine for several months. During the course of the consultation she continues to scratch her abdomen. Liver function tests: bilirubin 57 µmol/l, alkaline phosphatase 556 iu/litre normal aspartate aminotransferase and alanine aminotransferase. A liver biopsy shows expansion of the portal tracts by lymphocytes, plasma cells and occasional granulomas. Bile ducts are scarce.

67 THEME: DISORDERS OF THE PANCREAS

A Acute pancreatitis
B Adenocarcinoma of the pancreas
C β-cell tumour of the pancreas
D Chronic pancreatitis
E Cystic fibrosis
F Type I diabetes
G Type II diabetes
H Vipoma
I Zollinger–Ellison syndrome

The following are all descriptions of pancreatic disorders. Please select the most appropriate diagnosis from the list above. The items may be used once, more than once, or not at all.

☐ **1** A 27-year-old man presents with a 7-day history of abdominal pain, which radiates through to the back. He has been vomiting continuously over the past 2 days and has not been able to keep any fluid down. His bowels are open regularly with no history of steatorrhoea. There is no history of any similar episodes in the past. On examination he is pale, dehydrated and in considerable pain. He has marked epigastric peritonism on abdominal examination. Serum biochemistry includes; glucose 6.5 mmol/litre, urea 9.3 mmol/litre, creatinine 95 μmol/litre, corrected calcium 2.00, amylase 89.

☐ **2** A 52-year-old woman presents with a long history of intermittent diarrhoea, which has now become acute. Over the past 2 weeks she has passed watery stools up to ten times a day. This has left her feeling generally weak and she complains of generalised muscular cramps. She is not on any medication. Of note, her serum potassium is 2.8.

☐ **3** A 36-year-old man presents with repeated fainting and feeling light-headed. This seems to occur at irregular intervals and is most noticeable in the morning and during exercise. His general practitioner initially thought he might have a duodenal ulcer as he had been complaining of vague abdominal pain at night, which was relieved by eating. On examination he is pale, sweating and appears distracted. In addition, his hands are trembling.

68 THEME: SCORING IN ACUTE PANCREATITIS

A APACHE II
B Balthazar–Ranson grading system
C Computed tomography severity index
D Glasgow score = 2
E Glasgow score = 3
F Glasgow score = 4
G Hong Kong scoring
H Ranson score = 2
I Ranson score = 3
J Ranson score = 4
K Ranson score = 5

The above are examples of scores or scoring systems used in the early assessment of acute pancreatitis. From the descriptions below please choose the most appropriate answer from the list above. Each item may be used once, more than once, or not at all.

☐ **1** A 50-year-old woman with known gallstone disease presents to The Emergency Department one morning complaining of gnawing epigastric pain that radiates through to her back. Bloods on admission were amylase 950 iu/litre; full blood count: haemoglobin 12.4 g/dl, white cell count 17.2 × 10^9/litre, platelets 300 × 10^9/litre, haematocrit 0.38; glucose 7.8; lactate dehydrogenase 300 units/litre; liver function tests: albumin 38 g/litre, γ-glutamyltransferase 27 units/litre, aspartate aminotransferase 30 iu/litre, alkaline phosphatase 200; urea 6.4. Forty-eight hours later further tests are undertaken: full blood count: haemoglobin 11.9 g/dl, white cell count 18.2 × 10^9/litre, platelets 320 × 10^9/litre, haematocrit 0.25; liver function tests: albumin 34 g/litre, γ-glutamyltransferase 29 units/litre, aspartate aminotransferase 38, alkaline phosphatase 250; blood gases: $p_A(O_2)$ 10.4 kPa, base deficit −4.2; urea 7.4, Ca^{2+} 2.20.

☐ **2** A 58-year-old woman with a prior history of acute pancreatitis presents with symptoms similar to her previous attack. Her amylase is 920. Full blood count: haemoglobin 13.4 g/dl, white cell count 10.2 × 10^9/litre, platelets 300 × 10^9/litre; glucose 7.8, lactate dehydrogenase 300; liver function tests: albumin 37, γ-glutamyltransferase 18, aspartate aminotransferase 115, alkaline phosphatase 320; urea 6.1, Ca^{2+} 2.25.

☐ **3** A radiological scoring system that assesses pancreatic size, inflammation and fluid collections; that does not use intravenous contrast.

69 THEME: COMPLICATIONS OF GALLSTONE DISEASE

A Acute cholecystitis
B Acute pancreatitis
C Ascending cholangitis
D Biliary colic
E Chronic cholecystitis
F Empyema of the gallbladder
G Gallbladder perforation
H Gallstone ileus
I Mirizzi's syndrome
J Mucocoele
K Obstructive jaundice

The following are descriptions of patients with complications of gallstone disease. Please select the most appropriate diagnosis from the above list. The items may be used once, more than once, or not at all.

☐ **1** A 72-year-old woman presents with severe colicky central abdominal pain and vomiting. On examination there is right upper quadrant tenderness, negative Murphy's sign, abdominal distension and tinkling bowel sounds. Blood results: total bilirubin 12 μmol/litre, aspartate aminotransferase 25 iu/litre, alanine aminotransferase 29 iu/litre, alkaline phosphatase 200 iu/litre, amylase 38 iu/litre; white cell count 8.0×10^9/litre.

☐ **2** A 63-year-old man presents with a 5-day history of severe upper abdominal pain and vomiting. On examination there is a profound tachypnoea and tachycardia; he has generalised upper abdominal tenderness.

70 THEME: MANAGEMENT OF GALLSTONE DISEASE

A Endoscopic Retrograde Cholangio-Pancreatogram (ERCP) and sphincterotomy
B Early laparoscopic cholecystectomy +/− pre-operative cholangiography
C Interval laparoscopic cholecystectomy +/− pre-operative cholangiography
D Laparoscopic cholecystectomy + common bile duct exploration
E Laparotomy with cholecystotomy/drainage
F Magnetic resonance cholangiopancreatogram (MRCP)
G Open cholecystectomy + common bile duct exploration
H Non-surgical treatment, eg chemical dissolution therapy
I Percutaneous (radiological) gallbladder drainage

The following scenarios describe patients suffering from a complication of gallstone disease. From the above list, choose the single most appropriate definitive management option. Each item may be used once, more than once, or not at all.

☐ **1** A 45-year-old woman presents with a 2-day history of right upper quadrant pain, rigors, nausea and vomiting. She is febrile and her sclerae are noted to be yellow. Abdominal examination reveals a tender right hypochondrium. Liver function tests: bilirubin 29 μmol/l, alkaline phosphatase 450, aspartate aminotransferase 25 iu/litre. Ultrasound demonstrates a common bile duct diameter of 8 mm with multiple stones present.

☐ **2** A 35-year-old woman presents with worsening pain in her right upper quadrant associated with nausea and vomiting. She is neither clinically nor biochemically jaundiced but is febrile. An ultrasound reveals gallstones, thickening of the gallbladder wall and a common bile duct diameter of 3 mm.

☐ **3** A 79-year-old man presents with a 5-day history of progressive right upper quadrant pain. On examination, he is clearly septic. Examination reveals a very tender mass in the left upper quadrant. White cell count 21×10^9/litre.

71 THEME: RECTAL BLEEDING

A Anal carcinoma
B Anal fissure
C Angiodysplasia
D Colonic carcinoma
E Colonic polyp
F Crohn's disease
G Diverticular disease
H Haemorrhoids
I Infective colitis
J Ischaemic colitis
K Peri-anal haematoma
L Peptic ulceration
M Ulcerative colitis

The following patients have all presented with rectal bleeding. Please select the most appropriate diagnosis from the above list. The items may be used once, more than once, or not at all.

☐ **1** A 61-year-old renal transplant patient is referred to you on-call with acute-onset severe bloody diarrhoea. He appears clinically very unwell. He has no history of bowel problems.

☐ **2** A 27-year-old woman is seen with a 3-day history of acute diarrhoea which she attributes to food-poisoning. Today she has attended because of fresh rectal bleeding on the paper after wiping and once in the pan, separate from the stool.

☐ **3** A 92-year-old woman presents with painless, bright-red rectal bleeding without other symptoms. Following a blood transfusion a barium enema is performed, the result of which is normal, and she is sent back to the nursing home. One week later, she rebleeds and returns to The Emergency Department. Again the bleeding settles, and after re-transfusion, she undergoes a gastroscopy and colonoscopy at which no abnormality is detected.

72 THEME: CONSTIPATION

A Colorectal carcinoma
B Constipation-predominant irritable bowel syndrome
C Diabetes mellitus
D Eating disorders
E Functional faecal retention
F Hirschsprung's disease
G Hypercalcaemia
H Hypothyroidism
I Iatrogenic drug therapy
J Idiopathic megabowel
K Idiopathic 'slow-transit' constipation
L Neurogenic constipation
M Pelvic nerve injury
N Outlet obstruction
O Severe depression
P Simple constipation

The following patients all present with constipation. From the list above, select the most likely diagnosis. The items may be used once, more than once, or not at all.

☐ **1** A 53-year-old woman presents with a 2-year history of increasing difficulty passing stool. She currently opens her bowels daily or on alternate days. However, she has to strain excessively and often has to press on her perineum to achieve evacuation. She also reports a 'bulge' in the vagina when she gets constipated. She has attended clinic for the results of her recent investigations. Blood investigations and colonoscopy were normal.

☐ **2** A 74-year-old man presents to the surgical clinic with a 2-month history of constipation. Previously, he opened his bowels daily, passing stool of 'normal' consistency, but his bowels have become irregular, and he has experienced episodes of 'diarrhoea' during the last few weeks. On direct questioning, he reported episodic fresh bleeding per rectum, which he attributed to his 'piles'.

☐ **3** A 22-year-old man with a history of constipation since early childhood attends The Emergency Department having not opened his bowels for the previous 3 weeks. He was admitted with similar symptoms several months ago, when a rectal biopsy was performed. This demonstrated normal ganglion cells in the myenteric plexus, and no other abnormality. On examination he appears well. Abdominal examination reveals a large mass arising in the pelvis and extending to the umbilicus.

73 THEME: DIARRHOEA

A Amoebic dysentery
B Bacterial enterocolitis
C Colonic carcinoma
D Crohn's disease
E Diabetes
F Irritable bowel disease
G Giardiasis
H Malabsorption
I Neuro-endocrine tumour
J Overflow (faecal impaction)
K Pancreatic exocrine insufficiency
L Pseudomembranous colitis
M Thyrotoxicosis
N Ulcerative colitis

The following scenarios describe patients with diarrhoea. From the above list choose the most appropriate cause. Each item may be used once, more than once, or not at all.

☐ **1** A 35-year-old woman presents with a 1-month history of passing bloody diarrhoea/mucus up to seven times per day and lower abdominal pain. She was previously fit and well and her problems started following an episode of food poisoning in Thailand. She has associated lethargy and weight loss. On examination, she appears pale and abdominal examination reveals some lower abdominal tenderness. Haemoglobin 9.8 g/dl, mean corpuscular volume 60, white cell count 13 $\times$ 10^9/litre, erythrocyte sedimentation rate 65, C-reactive protein 130. A stool culture is negative. Sigmoidoscopy demonstrates active proctitis.

☐ **2** A 24-year-old man presents to clinic with a few months of diarrhoea and abdominal pain. At colonoscopy, there is patchy active inflammation affecting the transverse and right colon. Biopsies are reported as indeterminate colitis.

74 THEME: TYPES OF COLITIS

A Collagenous colitis
B Crohn's colitis
C Diversion colitis
D Infective colitis
E Ischaemic colitis
F Lymphocytic colitis
G Pseudomembranous colitis
H Radiation colitis
I Ulcerative colitis

The following patients have all been referred by their general practitioners with possible colitis. Please select the most appropriate diagnosis from the above list. The items may be used once, more than once, or not at all.

☐ **1** A 47 year-old woman with long-standing diabetes is seen with a 6-month history of colicky lower abdominal pain and watery diarrhoea. Her symptoms are intermittent; however, during 'attacks' she finds that she may open her bowel up to seven times a day with the passage of watery diarrhoea. These episodes are associated with lower abdominal pain and leave her feeling dehydrated and weak. So far she has had multiple blood tests, including erythrocyte sedimentation rate and C-reactive protein, which are normal. A colonoscopy is arranged which demonstrates a macroscopically normal looking colonic and terminal ileal mucosa. An OGD demonstrates duodenal villous atrophy.

☐ **2** A 77-year-old man is seen in The Emergency Department with a 1-day history of sudden onset of severe lower abdominal pain, vomiting and passage of bloody diarrhoea. On examination he is pyrexial (temperature 38 °C), tachycardic (pulse 105/min) and hypotensive (blood pressure 85/46 mmHg). He has severe left-sided tenderness and guarding on abdominal examination.

☐ **3** A 47-year-old man is referred for elective colectomy. You catch the end of the pathology discussion, which concludes that he has DALMs (Dysplasia-associated lesion or mass).

75 THEME: INVESTIGATION OF DISORDERS OF THE LARGE INTESTINE

A Abdominal radiograph
B Anorectal physiology
C Barium enema
D Colonoscopy
E Computed tomography scan of chest, abdomen and pelvis
F Examination under anaesthesia
G Flexible sigmoidoscopy
H Laparoscopy
I Laparotomy
J Mesenteric angiography
K Magnetic resonance imaging of pelvis
L Proctoscopy
M Water-soluble contrast enema
N Ultrasound scan of liver

The following patients have all presented with disorders of the large intestine. Please select the next most appropriate investigative step in the management. The items may be used once, more than once, or not at all.

☐ **1** A 52-year-old woman is seen in the outpatient department. She has no specific complaints herself but is worried as her sister, who is 43 years old, has been diagnosed with an adenocarcinoma of the sigmoid. There is no other family history of note.

☐ **2** A 54-year-old man is seen in the clinic for follow-up. He initially presented with rectal bleeding. Proctoscopy and rigid sigmoidoscopy performed at the time revealed a 1-cm benign-looking polyp, 15 cm from the anal verge, which was biopsied. The histology report reads ‘fragments of a moderately dysplastic villous adenoma’.

☐ **3** An 86-year-old woman is admitted to hospital with a history of sudden onset of severe rectal bleeding. She has been resuscitated but continues to bleed. An OGD has been performed, which is normal, and a colonoscopy is performed which demonstrates the presence of a large volume of blood in the lumen of the bowel. The endoscopist is unable to define the source of bleeding because of the view being obscured by active bleeding which could not be aspirated. She is currently stable, blood pressure 120/65 mmHg, pulse 85/min, and is receiving her fifth unit of blood.

☐ **4** A 49-year-old man is referred with a history of weight loss and anaemia. He has undergone a flexible sigmoidoscopy, which demonstrated a friable, annular constricting tumour in the descending colon. the endoscopist was unable to examine the colon proximal to this lesion. The histology, from biopsies taken, demonstrates adenocarcinoma.

☐ **5** A 63-year-old man is seen in The Emergency Department with a 4-day history of colicky lower abdominal pain, absolute constipation and distension. On direct questioning he admits to recent weight loss and rectal bleeding. On examination his abdomen is distended but soft. Plain radiography demonstrates large bowel distension.

76 THEME: FAECAL INCONTINENCE

A Colorectal carcinoma
B Dementia
C Extra-rectal or rectovaginal fistula
D Faecal impaction
E Inflammatory bowel disease
F Pudendal neuropathy
G Sphincter disruption
H Spinal cord lesion
I Systemic neuropathology

The following patients have all presented with faecal incontinence. From the above list choose the most appropriate cause. Each item may be used once, more than once, or not at all.

☐ **1** A 26-year-old woman is referred from her general practitioner with passive faecal incontinence following the birth of her child 3 months ago.

☐ **2** A 68-year-old man presents with new onset of faecal incontinence. He has been previously fit and well but now describes passing loose stools with an increased frequency.

☐ **3** A 60-year-old woman with four children presents with a 3-year history of worsening urge faecal incontinence. She had two prolonged, instrumented deliveries.

77 THEME: FISTULA-IN-ANO (CLASSIFICATION)

A Extrasphincteric
B High transsphincteric
C Intersphincteric
D Low transsphincteric
E Mid-transsphincteric
F Submucosal
G Suprasphincteric

The following are descriptions of fistula-in-ano. Please select the most appropriate anatomical description from the list. The items may be used once, more than once, or not at all.

☐ **1** A 34-year-old man is undergoing an examination under anaesthesia for long-standing fistula-in ano. The operating surgeon notes that the internal opening is at the level of the dentate line, with the fistula thence traversing both sphincters to an external opening 4 cm from the anal verge.

☐ **2** A 42-year-old man is referred to the outpatient clinic for a 7-month history of recurrent peri-anal pain and swelling followed by discharge of purulent fluid. Examination reveals a small opening, 1 cm from the anal verge. Palpation of the surrounding tissue suggests an indurated tract, passing from the opening through the internal anal sphincter to the dentate line. It does not seem to traverse the external anal sphincter.

☐ **3** A 28-year-old woman with extensive peri-anal Crohn's disease, continuously experiences peri-anal discharge of sero-sanguinous fluid following drainage of an ischiorectal abscess. STIR-sequence magnetic resonance imaging scans reveals a tract passing through the ischiorectal fossa and levator ani directly into the rectum.

78 THEME: TREATMENT OF BENIGN ANORECTAL DISORDERS

A Barrier cream
B Botulinum toxin injection
C Diltiazem ointment
D Drainage seton
E Fistulotomy
F Formaldehyde therapy
G Glycerol trinitrate ointment
H Haemorrhoidectomy
I Incision and drainage
J Injection sclerotherapy
K Lateral internal anal sphincterotomy
L Mapping excisional biopsy
M Prednisolone enema
N Rubber-band ligation

The following patients have all presented with symptoms of an anorectal disorder. Please select the most appropriate treatment from the above list. The items may be used once, more than once, or not at all.

☐ **1** A 37-year-old man presents with a 6-month history of intermittent peri-anal pain and swelling followed by purulent discharge; he is fully continent. A later examination under anaesthesia reveals a fistulous tract, commencing at the dentate line, following an inter-sphincteric course.

☐ **2** A 19-year-old woman presents with a 2-month history of pain and fresh bleeding on defaecation; her past medical history includes cluster headaches. Examination reveals a peri-anal sentinel skin tag at the 12 o'clock position; proctoscopy cannot be performed because of patient discomfort.

☐ **3** A 62-year-old woman presents 3 months after repeat injection sclerotherapy of haemorrhoids with an ongoing history of passing fresh blood per rectum, and the sensation of a lump coming down which she manually reduces. On examination, she has significant prolapsing haemorrhoids.

79 THEME: DISEASES OF THE ANUS

A Anal carcinoma
B Anal intra-epithelial neoplasia
C Anal fissure
D Anal fistula
E Condylomata acuminata
F Fibroepithelial anal polyp
G Haemorrhoids
H Peri-anal abscess
I Peri-anal haematoma
J Pilonidal abscess
K Proctalgia fugax
L Skin tags
M Solitary rectal ulcer syndrome

The following are descriptions of local anorectal disorders. Please select the most appropriate diagnosis from the list. The items may be used once, more than once, or not at all.

☐ **1** A 24-year-old man presents with a 3-month history of pain and passage of fresh blood on defaecation. Examination reveals a small skin tag at the anal verge; attempted proctoscopy has to be abandoned because of patient discomfort.

☐ **2** A condition associated with chronic infection with human papillomavirus (especially serotypes 16 and 18).

☐ **3** A 31-year-old man presents with a 1-year history of severe anal pain lasting for 2 to 3 minutes each night. Per rectum and proctosigmoidoscopic examinations are unremarkable.

Breast/endocrine surgery

80 THEME: BREAST LUMPS

A	Breast abscess	G	Lipoma
B	Breast cyst	H	Lobular carcinoma
C	Fibroadenoma	I	Peri-ductal mastitis
D	Fibrosarcoma	J	Phylloides tumour
E	Galactocoele	K	Sebaceous cyst
F	Invasive ductal carcinoma	L	Traumatic fat necrosis

The above are all potential causes of a lump in the breast. For the following clinical scenarios please select the most appropriate answer from the list. Items may be used once, more than once, or not at all.

☐ **1** A 28-year-old woman presents to Casualty complaining of right breast tenderness and redness with a recently enlarging swelling next to the nipple. She has been breastfeeding her newborn baby and thought initially that the redness was just soreness from a cracked nipple. On examination there is a tense peri-areolar swelling in the upper, outer quadrant of the right breast.

☐ **2** A 20-year-old woman presents to the breast clinic via her general practitioner. She tells you that she has recently noticed a smooth, small lump in her right breast. On examination there is a 1.5-cm, well-defined, mobile lump in the lower outer quadrant of the breast. She has no palpable lymph nodes. Fine-needle aspiration cytology (FNAC) comes back as C2 and ultrasonography confirms a discrete, solid lesion with clear margins and no acoustic shadow.

☐ **3** A 48-year-old woman presents to the breast outpatient clinic. She has recently noticed a painful lump in her left breast which has increased in size over the past week. On examination you note a tense swelling within the substance of the breast. Just larger than 2 cm in size, it has a smooth surface. There is no axillary lymphadenopathy. FNAC reveals greenish fluid and ultrasonography after this procedure cannot identify any clear lesion.

☐ **4** A 57-year-old woman presents to the one-stop breast clinic. She had noticed a firm lump in her right breast several months prior but had been reluctant to see her general practitioner because of embarrassment. Examining her you notice a firm lump in the upper outer quadrant of her right breast. It is large and has an irregular surface. You notice that the skin does not move freely over the swelling and she has some palpable lymph nodes in her right axilla. FNAC comes back as C5 and her mammogram shows regions of branching microcalcification. The other breast feels normal.

81 THEME: MASTALGIA

A Acute mastitis
B Aberrations of normal development and involution (ANDI)
C Breast abscess
D Breast carcinoma
E Cyclical mastalgia
F Fat necrosis
G Fibroadenosis
H Mondor's disease
I Tietze's syndrome

The following patients have presented to the one-stop breast clinic with mastalgia. Please select the most appropriate dignosis from the list above. The items may be used once, more than once, or not at all.

☐ **1** A 33-year-old woman is seen with a 1-day history of painful enlargement of her right breast. Of note, she is currently breast-feeding and is a smoker. On examination she has generalised enlargement of her right breast. The overlying skin is erythematous, hot to touch and tender. There are no masses palpable. Breast ultrasound is normal.

☐ **2** A 27-year-old woman presents with a 6-month history of intermittent pain along the inner aspect of her left brerast. The pain occurs for a few days before resolving spontaneously. The frequency of 'attacks' is increasing. She is an amateur athlete and complains that the pain prevents her from taking part in any physical activity. Breast examination is unremarkable apart from some tenderness medially.

☐ **3** A 58 year-old woman presents with a 2-week history of a mild ache and prickling sensation in her right breast. She is worried as she thinks she can now feel a lump in the area of concern. She has had a previous hysterectomy and bilateral salpingo-oophorectomy at the age of 45 and has been on hormone replacement therapy since. There is no family history of breast disease. On examination a non-tender, hard lump is palpable in the upper outer quadrant of the right breast.

82 THEME: NIPPLE DISCHARGE

A Breast carcinoma
B Epithelial hyperplasia
C Fibrocystic disease
D Intraductal carcinoma
E Mammary duct ectasia
F Mammary duct fistula
G Mammary intraductal papilloma
H Peri-ductal mastitis
I Physiological
J Prolactinoma

The following scenarios describe patients presenting with nipple discharge. From the above list of possible causes, choose the most likely diagnosis. Each answer may be chosen once, more than once, or not at all.

☐ **1** A 55-year-old lady presents with a 2-month history of 'cheesy' nipple discharge. On examination her breast is tender, and her nipple is retracted. You are able to express discharge from multiple ducts, which tests positive with Haemo-Stix. Mammography on the left shows some coarse calcification behind the nipple.

☐ **2** A 60-year-old lady is re-called following a screening mammogram that demonstrates a dilated retro-areolar duct. She recalls a brief episode 3 months previously of blood-stained nipple discharge that you are able to reproduce clinically. Her breast examination is otherwise normal.

☐ **3** A 49-year-old man presents with a watery, occasionally purulent nipple discharge that has been worsening over the last 6 months. He is a smoker. On examination there is marked peri-areolar inflammation and a fluctuant area lateral to the affected nipple.

☐ **4** A 45-year-old woman with a family history of breast cancer presents with a 3-week history of blood-stained nipple discharge. She reports that it is consistently produced from the same small area on her right nipple. On examination you concur, but otherwise there are no other notable findings. Fine-needle aspirate is reported as suspicious and mammography reveals fine microcalcification.

83 THEME: GYNAECOMASTIA

A Adrenocortical carcinoma
B Chronic liver disease
C Chronic renal failure
D Genetic
E Hyperthyroidism
F Iatrogenic drug therapy
G Hypogonadism
H Physiological
I Testicular tumour

The following patients all present with gynaecomastia. From the list above, select the most likely diagnosis. The items may be used once, more than once, or not at all.

☐ **1** A 23-year-old man is referred to clinic for assessment of gynaecomastia. He tells you that he remembers being conscious of the problem since childhood. Review of symptoms reveals that he has problems with his sense of smell. Past history includes maxillofacial surgery for a cleft lip and palate.

☐ **2** A 74-year-old man has been referred urgently by his general practitioner (GP) with a short history of bilateral breast swelling. The GP is concerned whether he might have a 'familial cancer syndrome' as he has recently been diagnosed with prostate cancer. The GP asks for your urgent opinion, since his prostate cancer was not detected early enough to allow surgical intervention.

☐ **3** A 38-year-old man with a 20-year history of type I diabetes on examination is found to have multiple scars on both forearms, and in the sub-umbilical region.

84 THEME: MANAGEMENT OF BREAST CANCER

A Anastrozole
B Axillary clearance
C Chemotherapy
D Excision of margins
E Mastectomy
F Radiotherapy
G Tamoxifen
H Wide local excision
I Wide local excision and axillary clearance
J Wire-guided wide local excision

The following descriptions are of patients with breast cancer. Please select the most appropriate treatment option. The items may be used once, more than once, or not at all.

☐ **1** A 57-year-old has been seen for follow-up with a history of a 2-cm lump in the upper outer quadrant of the right breast. Mammography and ultrasound are highly suspicious for breast cancer (R5, U5) and this is confirmed on fine-needle aspiration cytology (FNAC; C5) and core biopsy, which demonstrates invasive ductal carcinoma. Subsequent investigations reveal no evidence of metastatic disease.

☐ **2** A 45-year-old woman is seen following mastectomy and axillary clearance. She has made an uneventful recovery. The final histology report states 'invasive ductal carcinoma, completely excised with two out of 17 lymph nodes demonstrating infiltration with tumour. Oestrogen and progesterone receptor negative'. She asks you what further treatment is required.

☐ **3** A 53-year-old woman is seen in the clinic for results of biopsies from a screen-detected lesion in her right breast. Cytology from an FNA is graded as C4 and core biopsies have demonstrated the presence of intermediate grade ductal carcinoma *in situ* (DCIS).

☐ **4** An 89-year-old lady has been brought to the one-stop clinic by her daughter who noted a lump in her mother's left breast while dressing her. Her mother is wheelchair-bound, suffers with dementia and is normally a resident of a nursing home. On examination the patient is a frail woman with a large mass in the upper outer quadrant of her left breast. The mass is fixed to the skin and underlying muscle and, in addition, she has fixed lymph nodes in her left axilla. Core biopsies demonstrate an invasive ductal carcinoma, which is oestrogen and progesterone receptor positive.

☐ **5** A 45-year-old woman has undergone a wide local excision and axillary clearance for invasive ductal carcinoma. The final histology reads 'invasive ductal carcinoma with 2-mm clearance from the nearest (lateral margin). There is no evidence of lymph node metastases. Oestrogen and progesterone receptor negative'.

85 THEME: MISCELLANEOUS DISORDERS OF THE FEMALE BREAST

A Absence of breast tissue
B Accessory breast tissue
C Cystosarcoma phylloides
D Idiopathic benign breast hypertrophy
E Lipoma
F Lobular mastitis
G Mondor's disease
H Peri-ductal mastitis
I Sclerosing adenosis
J Traumatic fat necrosis
K Tuberculosis of the breast

The following scenario describes presentation of a woman with breast pathology. From the list above, choose the single most appropriate diagnosis. Each item may be used once, more than once, or not at all.

☐ **1** A 55-year-old woman complains of a 2-day history of pain in her right breast. The pain is described as localised to the lateral aspect of the breast and of sudden onset. She has no significant risk factors for breast cancer; however, she is extremely anxious. On examination she has a tender, subcutaneous, linear cord in the right breast. The overlying skin is acutely inflamed and becomes puckered on raising the right arm. Mammography and breast ultrasound are unremarkable.

86 THEME: THYROID SWELLINGS

A Anaplastic carcinoma
B De Quervain's thyroiditis
C Follicular adenoma
D Follicular carcinoma
E Graves' disease
F Haemorrhage into a cyst
G Hashimoto's thyroiditis
H Hyperplastic (colloid) goitre
I Lymphoma
J Medullary carcinoma
K Multinodular goitre
L Papillary carcinoma
M Riedel's thyroiditis

The above are all causes of a swelling within the thyroid gland. For each clinical scenario please pick the most appropriate answer from the list. The items may be used once, more than once, or not at all.

☐ **1** A 74-year-old woman presents with a history of a rapidly enlarging swelling in the left side of her neck. She tells you that swallowing is uncomfortable and sometimes food sticks at the top of her throat. On examination she has a diffuse, irregular swelling in the left lobe of her thyroid gland. The overlying skin has a slight red–blue tinge. You think that you can feel some ipsilateral lymphadenopathy on examination of the cervical glands. Thyroid function test: thyroid-stimulating hormone 4.2 mU/litre, free thyroxine 18.4 nmol/litre.

☐ **2** An 18-year-old woman presents to the surgical endocrine clinic on referral from her general practitioner. She complains of a small lump in the right side of her neck, which appears to be slowly enlarging. On examination you note a smooth, well-defined 1.5-cm nodule in the right thyroid lobe. There is a firm palpable lymph node present in the right anterior triangle. Thyroid function test: thyroid-stimulating hormone 5.2 mU/litre, free thyroxine 14.3 nmol/litre.

☐ **3** A 24-year-old woman is brought into The Emergency Department by her concerned boyfriend. She has laboured breathing with stridor. Her partner tells you that she has had a long-standing swelling in the neck which had always been inconsequential. However, earlier that day she had complained of sudden pain in the anterior neck. Thyroid function test: thyroid-stimulating hormone 3.9 mU/litre, free thyroxine 17.2 nmol/litre.

87 THEME: DISEASES OF THE THYROID GLAND

A Carcinoma of the thyroid
B Chronic lymphocytic thyroiditis
C De Quervain's thyroiditis
D Follicular adenoma
E Graves' disease
F Hashimoto's thyroiditis
G Lymphoma
H Multinodular goitre
I Myxoedema coma
J Primary myxoedema
K Riedel's thyroiditis
L Sick euthyroidism
M Simple colloid goitre
N Struma ovarii
O Thyroid storm
P Toxic adenoma

The following scenarios describe patients with a thyroid condition. From the list above, choose the most likely diagnosis. Each item may be chosen once, more than once, or not at all. The normal range for tri-iodothyronine (T_3) is 1.2–3.0 nmol/litre, for thyroxine (T_4) it is 70–140 nmol/litre and for thyroid stimulating hormone (TSH) it is 0.5–5.7 mU/litre.

☐ **1** A 25-year-old man presents with a 3-week history of passing loose stools and is noted to have a slight resting tremor and a pulse rate of 90/min. He recalls recently feeling unwell with a sore throat and sinusitis. On examination his thyroid is soft, tender and bilaterally enlarged. His thyroid function tests are normal and a scintiscan shows low thyroid uptake.

☐ **2** A 45-year-old man is ventilated following laparotomy for a peritonitis secondary to gangrenous appendicitis. His condition has been deteriorating and recent thyroid function tests reveal a T_3 of 8 nmol/litre, T_4 of 190 nmol/litre and TSH of 2 mU/litre.

88 THEME: COMPLICATIONS OF THYROIDECTOMY

A Air embolism
B Haemorrhage
C Bilateral complete recurrent laryngeal nerve paralysis
D Bilateral incomplete recurrent laryngeal nerve paralysis
E Hypocalcaemia
F Hypothyroidism
G Superior laryngeal nerve paralysis
H Pneumothorax
I Recurrent hyperthyroidism
J Thyroid crisis
K Tracheal collapse
L Unilateral complete recurrent laryngeal nerve paralysis
M Unilateral incomplete recurrent laryngeal nerve paralysis
N Thyroid storm

The following are descriptions of patients post-thyroidectomy. Please select the most appropriate diagnosis from the above list. The items may be used once, more than once, or not at all.

☐ **1** A 27-year-old woman 2 days post-thyroidectomy has numbness around the mouth and the sensation of 'pins and needles' in her fingers.

☐ **2** A 50-year-old woman becomes acutely confused 12 h post-thyroidectomy. She has been complaining of severe abdominal pain, palpitations and diarrhoea. An electrocardiogram demonstrates atrial fibrillation.

☐ **3** A 45-year-old woman returns to outpatients 3 months after thyroidectomy. She complains that her vocal range appears diminished when she participates in her local amateur dramatics productions.

☐ **4** A 64-year-old man develops severe difficulty breathing shortly after a total thyroidectomy. Examination reveals respiratory rate 34 breaths/min and auscultation demonstrates inspiratory stridor. There is no neck swelling.

89 THEME: DISORDERS OF CALCIUM HOMEOSTASIS

A Acute pancreatitis
B Addison's disease
C Chronic renal failure
D Ectopic parathyroid hormone
E Familial hypocalciuric hypercalcaemia
F Hyperparathyroidism
G Hypoparathyroidism
H Malignancy
I Milk–alkali syndrome
J Multiple myeloma
K Osteomalacia
L Pseudohypoparathyroidism
M Sarcoidosis
N Thiazides
O Thyrotoxicosis
P Vitamin D deficiency

The following scenarios describe patients with disorders of calcium metabolism. Choose from the above list the most likely cause. Each item may be chosen once, more than once, or not at all.

☐ **1** A 45-year-old woman is 24 h post-parathyroidectomy and biopsy of her remaining gland. She complains of cramps in her hands and around her mouth. Her plasma calcium is 1.95 mmol/litre and serum albumin is 42 g/litre.

☐ **2** A 55-year-old woman is seen in the urology clinic after attending Casualty with recurrent stones. She comments that she is also undergoing treatment for peptic ulceration. Her history is unremarkable, and she is otherwise well and takes no other regular medication. Her plasma calcium is found to be 3.2 mmol/litre with an albumin of 47 g/litre.

☐ **3** A 65-year-old man presents with severe back pain and recurrent bleeding from his gums. He also mentions that his vision has become increasingly blurred in recent weeks. His plasma calcium is 2.95 mmol/litre.

90 THEME: CAUSES OF SECONDARY HYPERTENSION

A Acromegaly
B Adrenal hyperplasia
C Chronic pyelonephritis
D Coarctation of the aorta
E Conn's syndrome
F Cushing's syndrome
G Diabetes mellitus
H Glomerulonephritis
I Hyperparathyroidism
K Oral contraceptive pill
L Phaeochromocytoma
M Polyarteritis nodosa
N Polycystic kidneys
O Pre-eclampsia
P Renal artery stenosis
Q Renin-secreting tumours
R Steroid therapy
S Systemic sclerosis

The following scenarios describe various patients with secondary hypertension. From the list above choose the single most appropriate cause for their secondary hypertension. Each item may be chosen once, more than once, or not at all.

☐ **1** A 35-year-old woman presents to clinic with episodic headaches, sweating and palpitations. Her blood pressure is 205/100 mmHg and her 24-h urinary collection demonstrates elevated metanephrines.

☐ **2** A 26-year-old man presents with haematuria, recurrent episodes of non-specific abdominal pain and melaena. He often wakes up with night sweats and describes diffuse myalgia. He takes no regular medication and has a blood pressure of 195/90 mmHg.

☐ **3** A 45-year-old woman attends Casualty with muscular cramps and tetany, polyuria and nocturia. Her electrocardiogram demonstrates a prolonged PR interval and on questioning she describes occasional palpitations. She is noted to be hypertensive and takes no regular medication. Her potassium is 3.1 mmol/litre.

☐ **4** A 55-year-old man is due to undergo an inguinal hernia repair but in pre-assessment clinic is noted to have a blood pressure of 220/95 mmHg. On examination he has excessive fat deposition around the nape of his neck and multiple striae across his abdomen. He takes no regular medication.

Vascular surgery

91 THEME: THE PAINFUL LOWER LIMB

A Atherosclerosis
B Buerger's disease
C Chronic venous insufficiency
D Degenerative joint disease
E Deep venous thrombosis
F Embolus
G Polymyalgia rheumatica
H Polymyositis
I Raynaud's disease
J Ruptured Baker's cyst
K Sciatica
L Scleroderma
M Septic arthritis
N Superficial thrombophlebitis

From the list above, select the most likely diagnosis for the following patients who all present with pain in the lower limb. The items may be used once, more than once, or not at all.

☐ **1** A 32-year-old man with a long history of intravenous drug abuse attends The Emergency Department with a 4-h history of very severe pain in his left leg. On examination, the patient is in sinus rhythm. The limb is pale and cold compared to the other side, and only the femoral pulse is present. Pulses are normal contralaterally.

☐ **2** A 54-year-old woman is referred to clinic with limb pain. She describes a dull ache that is worse at the end of the day, and that affects the right side more than the left. She has a past history of deep venous thrombosis. On examination, varicose veins are evident in the distribution of the long sapheous system, and there is brown pigmentation of the skin of the lower third of both legs. There is also a small ulcer superior to the medial malleolus.

☐ **3** A 28-year-old man of Chinese origin with a history of calf pain induced by exercise presents to The Emergency Department with gangrene of the left great toe. He reports a history of preceding calf pain induced by exercise. He is a heavy smoker, but has no other risk factors for atherosclerosis. Examination reveals absent pedal pulses on the affected side.

92 THEME: ULCERATION IN THE LOWER LIMB

A Arteriovenous fistula
B Ischaemic ulcer
C Necrobiosis lipoidica
D Neoplastic ulcer
E Neuropathic ulcer
F Pyoderma gangrenosum
G Self-inflicted
H Sickle cell disease
I Syphilis
J Traumatic ulcer
K Tuberculosis
L Vasculitic ulcer
M Venous ulcer

The following scenarios describe patients with leg ulceration. From the above list of causes of ulceration, choose the most appropriate answer. Each item may be used once, more than once, or not at all.

☐ **1** A 55-year-old diabetic man presents with a large painless ulcer on the sole of his foot. On examination, the ulcer appears deep with healthy surrounding skin. The foot feels warm and his ankle-brachial pressure index is 0.8.

☐ **2** A 27-year-old man presents with abdominal pain, bloody diarrhoea and weight loss. On examination he is noted to have some areas of necrotising ulceration surrounded by erythema over his legs, which are acutely painful.

☐ **3** A 60-year-old lady presents with brown discoloration of both calves and a large left medial malleolar ulcer. A central raised patch of friable, irregular, nodular growth is noted.

93 THEME: THE SWOLLEN LOWER LIMB

A Angio-oedema
B Congestive cardiac failure
C Chronic renal failure
D Chronic liver failure
E Chronic venous insufficiency
F Deep venous thrombosis
G Factitious oedema
H Klippel–Trenaunay syndrome
I Malabsorption
J Malnutrition
K Milroy's disease
L Obesity
M Primary lymphoedema
N Secondary lymphoedema
O Venous obstruction

The following patients all present with swelling affecting the lower limb. From the list above, select the most likely diagnosis. The items may be used once, more than once, or not at all.

☐ **1** A 21-year-old woman is referred to clinic with a history of intermittent oedema of the face and extremities. Her mother also suffers with similar symptoms.

☐ **2** A 14-year-old boy is referred to clinic for assessment of varicose veins and associated swelling of his left leg. As he enters the consultation room you note that he has a 'short-leg' gait. His varicose veins are large and do not lie in a typical distribution.

☐ **3** A 48-year-old woman presents with a history of unilateral swelling of the right leg. There is no history of venous obstruction. Her general practitioner has sent copies of recent full blood counts, urea & electrolytes, and liver function tests, all of which are normal. Isotope lymphography demonstrates delayed transit of radionuclide on the right side.

94 THEME: MANAGEMENT OF PERIPHERAL VASCULAR DISORDERS

A Above-knee amputation
B Aortofemoral bypass
C Atherosclerosis risk factor reduction
D Below-knee amputation
E Femorodistal bypass
F Femorofemoral bypass
G Femoropopliteal bypass
H Intraluminal stenting
I Long saphenous vein surgery
J Percutaneous thrombolytic thromboembolectomy
K Percutaneous transluminal angioplasty
L Sclerotherapy
M Short saphenous vein surgery
N Surgical thromboembolectomy

The following are descriptions of patients with peripheral vascular disorders. Please select the most appropriate treatment from the above list. The items may be used once, more than once, or not at all.

☐ **1** A 57-year-old man presents with left-sided cramping calf pain after walking approximately 100 metres. Examination of both lower limbs reveals no significant abnormalities.

☐ **2** A 64-year-old man presents with sudden onset of severe left-sided calf pain. On examination his left foot is pale and cold; on the affected side he has no palpable pulses below the femoral pulse. He is currently recovering from a recent cerebrovascular accident.

☐ **3** A 37-year-old woman presents with prominent unsightly leg veins, which cause discomfort on prolonged standing. Examination reveals tortuous dilated subcutaneous veins along the medial aspect of the right calf; tourniquet tests indicate that when tied around the upper thigh and again just above the knee, the varicosities refill upon standing; however, when tied just below the knee they are controlled. She is currently taking oral contraception.

Transplant

95 THEME: COMPLICATIONS OF CADAVERIC ORGAN TRANSPLANTATION

A Acute rejection
B Arterial thrombosis
C Azathioprine side-effects
D Chronic rejection
E Cyclosporin side-effects
F Cytomegalovirus infection
G Graft-versus-host disease
H Hyperacute rejection
I Malignancy
J Primary graft non-function
K Steroid side-effects
L Venous thrombosis

The following patients have all previously undergone cadaveric organ transplantation. From the above list, select the most likely complication. The items may be used once, more than once, or not at all.

☐ **1** A 25-year-old woman with cystic fibrosis underwent a heart and lung transplant 4 months ago, and is currently receiving triple immunotherapy. She attends the follow-up clinic for a routine check-up. She reports sore gums and excessive facial hair. On examination she is hypertensive. Urea & electrolyte results are as follows: Na^+ 139 mmol/litre, K^+ 5.7 mmol/litre, urea 9.9 mmol/litre, creatinine 140 µmol/litre.

☐ **2** A 58-year-old man had a liver transplant 7 weeks ago. He attends The Emergency Department with a 24-h history of malaise, fever and myalgia and respiratory distress going upstairs. He is currently receiving triple immunosuppression. On examination, he is unwell and dyspnoeic at rest. He has a pulse rate of 105/min, blood pressure is 95/60 mmHg, temperature is 38.3 °C and respiratory rate is 28 breaths/min. Oxygen saturation is 90% on air.

☐ **3** A 41-year-old woman underwent renal transplantation 18 months ago. She attends follow-up clinic and is currently asymptomatic. On examination her blood pressure is 150/110 and urinalysis reveals 3^+ protein. Urine culture is negative. A renal ultrasound scan reveals a normal collecting system. Renal biopsy demonstrates intrarenal arteriosclerosis with associated glomerular atrophy and interstitial fibrosis.

Ear, nose and throat, and maxillofacial surgery

96 THEME: AUDITORY DISORDERS

- A Acoustic neuroma
- B Acute (serous) middle-ear effusion
- C Acute suppurative otitis media
- D Barotraumatic otitis media
- E Carcinoma of the middle ear and mastoid
- F Cholesteotoma
- G Chronic (serous) middle ear effusion
- H Chronic suppurative otitis media
- I Foreign body in the ear
- J Labyrinthitis
- K Ménière's disease
- L Otitis externa
- M Otosclerosis
- N Referred pain
- O Wax

The following patients have all presented with otalgia, discharge from the ear, or deafness. Please select the most appropriate diagnosis from the above list. The items may be used once, more than once, or not at all.

☐ **1** A 55-year-old man has been referred with a history of sudden onset of vertigo accompanied by nausea and vomiting that gradually subsided over 24 h but left him unsteady for 3 weeks. On direct questioning, he has noticed a hearing loss in his left ear and a period of tinnitus before the attack of vertigo. After the attack he noticed that his hearing had become worse. On examination, the only abnormal finding was a left-sided sensorineural hearing loss, confirmed on audiometry.

☐ **2** A 45-year-old man presents with a 1-year history of foul-smelling purulent discharge from the left ear and increasing deafness. On examination after removal of the discharge, an attic perforation is visualised which is occupied by a greyish substance. Radiography reveals a sclerotic mastoid.

☐ **3** A 20-year-old woman presents with a 1-year history of bilateral deafness and tinnitus. The deafness is worse on the left side and is less marked in places with background noise. The patient's father has worn a hearing aid since his late teens. On examination, the tympanic membranes are normal. Rinne's test is negative bilaterally, and Weber's test lateralises to the left side.

☐ **4** A 10-year-old child presents with rapid-onset, severe, right-sided otalgia and hearing loss following an upper respiratory tract infection. On examination, the right tympanic membrane appears red and bulges outwards

97 THEME: EPISTAXIS

A Chemical irritation
B Foreign body
C Haemophilia
D Hypertension
E Iatrogenic
F Idiopathic
G Malignant neoplasm
H Hereditary haemorrhagic telangectasia (Osler's disease)
I Pyogenic granuloma
J Rhinitis
K Thrombocytopaenia
L Trauma.
M Wegener's granuloma

The following patients have all presented with epistaxis. Please select the most appropriate diagnosis from the above list. The items may be used once, more than once, or not at all.

☐ **1** A 2-year-old child presents with bleeding from one side of the nose. His mother had noticed a foul-smelling discharge from the nose on that side for some months. This had only temporarily responded to courses of antibiotics. Examination of the nostrils shows an inflamed mucous membrane and a blood-stained mucopurulent discharge.

☐ **2** A 25-year-old man presents with a history of chronic sinusitis and epistaxis over the past 3 years. On rhinoscopy he has nasal crusting with a small septal defect. On oral examination there is quite marked gingivitis and tooth decay.

98 THEME: VOCAL PROBLEMS: DYSPHONIA

A Acute viral/bacterial laryngitis
B Candidiasis of the larynx
C Gastro-oesophageal reflux disease (GORD)
D Hypothyroidism
E Laryngeal carcinoma
F Laryngeal papilloma
G Neurogenic: left recurrent laryngeal nerve palsy
H Neurogenic: right recurrent laryngeal nerve palsy
I Neurogenic: superior laryngeal nerve palsy
J Neurogenic: vagal nerve palsy
K Singer's nodules
L Spasmodic dysphonia
M Trauma (external)
N Tuberculous laryngitis

The following patients have all presented with voice problems. Please select the most appropriate diagnosis from the above list. The items may be used once, more than once, or not at all.

☐ **1** A 28-year-old man reports hoarseness, especially in the morning. This resolves gradually during the day. There is no history of vocal abuse. He smokes 10 cigarettes a day and drinks moderately. On indirect laryngoscopy both cords are slightly red but there are no focal abnormalities.

☐ **2** A 60-year-old lifelong heavy smoker reports a rapid onset of hoarseness that has slightly improved while waiting for his Ear, Nose and Throat appointment. He has recently been investigated by the respiratory physicians for chronic cough with haemoptysis and weight loss. On examination he is clubbed.

☐ **3** A 5-year-old boy is brought to The Emergency Department with dyspnoea and stridor. His mother has noticed a change in his voice over the past 3 months. The general practitioner has been treating his progressive dyspnoea as asthma. On examination of the vocal cords there are multiple small pedunculated lesions on the vocal cords that are pinkish white in colour.

99 THEME: STRIDOR

A Acute epiglottitis
B Acute laryngotracheobronchitis
C Anaphylactic reaction
D Angioneurotic oedema
E Bilateral recurrent laryngeal nerve paralysis
F Carcinoma of the larynx
G Diphtheria
H Fracture of the larynx
I Inhaled foreign body
J Inhalation or ingestion of irritants
K Laryngeal papilloma
L Ludwig's angina
M Maxillofacial trauma
N Paralaryngeal haematoma
O Reduced consciousness level
P Thyroid carcinoma

The following patients have all presented with stridor. Please select the most appropriate diagnosis from the above list. The items may be used once, more than once, or not at all.

☐ **1** A 1-year-old child presents on Boxing Day with a mild upper respiratory tract infection that has progressively worsened. His mother now describes a cough like a seal's bark and stridor. The child has a temperature of 38.5 °C and is tachycardic. There is stridor and expiratory wheeze.

☐ **2** An 18-year-old girl presents with facial oedema, dyspnoea and stridor. She is apyrexial and has no past medical history, drug history, or allergies.

☐ **3** A 25-year-old fireman is rescued by his colleagues after becoming trapped by falling debris in a burning building. He is alert and orientated but has stridor, hoarseness and a cough productive of black sputum. He has burns to the face and upper torso.

100 THEME: NON-NEOPLASTIC SALIVARY GLAND DISEASE

A Acute suppurative sialadenitis
B HIV-associated sialadenitis
C Mikulicz's syndrome
D Sarcoidosis
E Sialolithiasis
F Sialosis
G Sjögren's syndrome
H Viral parotitis
I Xerostomia

From the list above, select the most likely diagnosis for the following patients who all present with disease affecting the salivary glands. The items may be used once, more than once, or not at all.

☐ **1** A 49-year-old man attends The Emergency Department with severe, sudden onset submandibular pain. Over the last few weeks he has experienced similar pain precipitated by eating, but never as severe as this. Past history includes hypertension. On examination, he is afebrile and there is diffuse submandibular swelling that is only minimally tender on bimanual palpation.

☐ **2** A 32-year-old woman is referred to clinic with parotidomegaly. She reports intermittent painless swelling over the last few months. Past medical history includes hypothyroidism and chronic back pain, for which she takes thyroxine 100 μg and co-proxamol, respectively. On examination, there is soft enlargement of the parotid gland.

☐ **3** A 50-year-old woman presents with a recent history of a dry mouth. On direct questioning she reports irritation of her eyes, although she denies arthralgia. There is no relevant past medical or drug history. Clinical examination of the salivary glands is unremarkable. Full blood count is normal, erythrocyte sedimentation rate and C-reactive protein are both grossly elevated.

101 THEME: SALIVARY GLAND TUMOURS

A Acinic cell carcinoma
B Adenocarcinoma
C Adenoid cystic carcinoma
D Epidermoid carcinoma
E Lymphoma
F Metastatic carcinoma
G Monomorphic adenoma (synonym: adenolymphoma – Warthin's tumour)
H Mucoepidermoid carcinoma
I Pleomorphic adenoma
J Squamous cell carcinoma

The following patients all present with salivary gland tumours. From the list above, select the most likely diagnosis. The items may be used once, more than once, or not at all.

☐ **1** A 47-year-old man is referred to clinic with unilateral swelling affecting the right parotid gland. He reports painless swelling, increasing in size over the last few years. Examination confirms intact facial nerve function, although inspection of the mouth reveals displacement of the right tonsil and pillar of the fauces towards the midline.

☐ **2** A 61-year-old woman has been referred urgently by her general practitioner with a history of painful swelling of the right parotid gland. She has recently developed facial nerve palsy on the right side. Examination reveals a cystic mass that is fixed over the parotid gland, and associated cervical lymphadenopathy. Fine-needle aspiration demonstrates the presence of atypical mucous cells.

☐ **3** A 71-year-old man presents with swelling of the left parotid gland. Examination reveals a non-tender enlargement of the left parotid gland, with bilateral cervical and axillary lymphadenopathy. There is intact facial nerve function. Full blood count: haemoglobin 8.8 g/dl, white cell count 2.2×10^9/litre, platelets 45×10^9/litre.

102 THEME: NECK LUMPS

A Branchial cyst
B Carotid body tumour
C Cervical rib
D Cystic hygroma
E Parotid tumour
F Pharyngeal pouch
G Sternocleidomastoid tumour
H Submandibular tumour
I Thyroglossal cyst
J Thyroid swellings
K Tonsillitis

The following scenarios describe various presentations of neck lumps. From the above list choose the most likely diagnosis. Each item may be chosen once, more than once, or not at all.

☐ **1** A 27-year-old man presents with a new lump in his neck that on examination is situated in the left carotid triangle, and appears to be deep to the upper third of the sternocleidomastoid muscle. It feels firm and cystic on palpation. Aspiration reveals 10 ml of thick yellow fluid. He is otherwise fit and well.

☐ **2** An 80-year-old woman presents with a history of dysphagia, halitosis, regurgitation and recurrent chest infections. She is otherwise well.

☐ **3** A 4-month-old infant is brought to clinic with a unilateral swelling on the right side of the neck. The child is noted to posture her head awkwardly. She is otherwise well but her mother reports that she was born by a difficult forceps delivery for a breech presentation.

☐ **4** A 20-year-old woman presents with an asymptomatic painless lump in the midline below her chin. The lump is smooth, measures 1 cm, is non tender and moves on swallowing.

103 THEME: ORAL/GLOSSAL LESIONS

A Carcinoma of the oral cavity
B Chronic superficial glossitis
C Fibroepithelial polyp
D Mucous retention cyst
E Pyogenic granuloma
F Ranula
G Stomatitis
H Sublingual dermoid cyst
I Thyroglossal cyst

From the list above, select the most likely diagnosis for the following patients who all present with lesions affecting the mouth. The items may be used once, more than once, or not at all.

☐ **1** A 31-year-old man attends The Emergency Department with a rapidly growing painless lump affecting the inside of the lower lip. He has just returned from a scuba-diving expedition in Australia 6 days ago.

☐ **2** A 26-year-old woman presents to clinic with a swelling 'underneath her tongue'. She reports a slight increase in size over the last few months. On examination, there is a soft, tense, translucent swelling in the floor of the mouth. There is no evidence of cervical lymphadenopathy.

☐ **3** A 62-year-old man presents with a painful, chronic ulcerating lesion in the left salivary gutter of the mouth. He has smoked 40 cigarettes per day for the last 50 years, and consumes approximately 30 units of alcohol each week.

104 THEME: CERVICAL LYMPHADENOPATHY

A Idiopathic histiocytic necrotising lymphadenitis
B Infectious mononucleosis
C Lymphoreticular disease
D Metastatic malignancy
E Sarcoidosis
F Scalp infection
G Tonsillitis
H Toxoplasmosis
I Tuberculosis

The following scenarios describe various presentations of cervical lymphadenopathy. From the above list choose the most likely cause. Each item may be chosen once, more than once, or not at all.

☐ **1** A 68-year-old man presents with an asymptomatic slowly growing painless lump in the neck. On examination he has a hard 2-cm mass lying laterally in the submandibular triangle of his neck, deep to the middle third of the right sternocleidomastoid muscle. The patient is noted to have a dysphonia.

☐ **2** A 12-year-old girl presents with recurrent sore throats and on examination she has a soft 2-cm mass lying laterally within the anterior triangle of the neck, just below the angle of the mandible.

☐ **3** A 28-year-old Caucasian presents with a 3-month history of night sweats, weight loss and a unilateral enlargement of his left tonsil. There is also a rubbery enlarged level III lymph node in the left posterior triangle.

Paediatric surgery

105 THEME: PAEDIATRIC SURGICAL DISORDERS

A	Acute appendicitis	H	Intussusception
B	Duodenal atresia	I	Malrotation
C	Duplication	J	Meconeum ileus
D	Hirschsprung's disease	K	Necrotising enterocolitis
E	Imperforate anus	L	Pyloric stenosis
F	Inguinal hernia	M	Septicaemia
G	Intestinal volvulus	N	Testicular torsion

The following are descriptions of paediatric surgical disorders. Please select the most appropriate diagnosis from the above list. The items may be used once, more than once or not at all.

☐ **1** A 1-day-old full-term infant presents with a 1-day history of abdominal distension and clear green vomiting; a sweat test reveals sodium and chloride levels >60 mmol/litre. Examination demonstrates upper abdominal distension. Plain abdominal radiograph shows a 'soap bubble' appearance in the right lower quadrant of the abdomen.

☐ **2** A 1-week-old pre-term infant presents with abdominal distension, green-stained vomit and bleeding per rectum. Examination demonstrates upper abdominal distension. Plain abdominal radiograph shows intramural intestinal gas.

☐ **3** A 9-month-old full-term infant presents with intermittent episodes of apparent abdominal pain, associated with vomiting and the passage of blood per rectum. Abdominal examination reveals a palpable sausage-shaped mass.

☐ **4** A 5-week-old full-term infant presents with a 1-day history of abdominal distension and clear projectile vomiting. Examination demonstrates a palpable 'olive-shaped' mass in the right upper quadrant.

Plastic surgery

106 THEME: MANAGEMENT OF BURNS

A 0.5–1 litres Ringer's lactate solution in 8 h
B 0.5–1 litres Ringer's lactate solution in 8 h, transfer to burns unit
C 1–2 litres Ringer's lactate solution in 8 h
D 1–2 litres Ringer's lactate solution in 8 h, transfer to burns unit
E 2–4 litres Ringer's lactate solution in 8 h
F 2–4 litres Ringer's lactate solution in 8 h, transfer to burns unit
G 3–6 litres Ringer's lactate solution in 8 h, transfer to burns unit
H 4–8 litres Ringer's lactate solution in 8 h, transfer to burns unit
I 5–10 litres Ringer's lactate solution in 8 h, transfer to burns unit

The following patients have all presented with burn injuries. Ignoring other measures (airway, breathing, intravenous access, dressings etc), please select the most appropriate fluid management plan from the above list. The items may be used once, more than once, or not at all. (BSA = body surface area.)

☐ **1** A 70-kg mechanical engineer sustains a mixture of partial and full thickness burns to his lower limbs (< 5% BSA, full-thickness) from a fractured pipe leaking pressurised steam. You calculate that he has 14% BSA total burns.

☐ **2** A 9-year-old child weighing 35 kg sustains 14% blistering burns to the upper limbs while trying to 'torch' a dumped car on his council estate.

☐ **3** A 27-year-old 70 kg man is rescued by the fire service from a house fire. He has extensive partial and full-thickness burns covering the front and back of the trunk and the front and back of one lower limb.

107 THEME: BENIGN SKIN AND SUBCUTANEOUS LESIONS

A Angioma
B Benign papilloma
C Clear cell acanthoma (viral warts)
D Epidermal cysts
E Ganglion
F Glomus tumour
G Histiocytoma
H Keratoacanthoma
I Lipoma
J Lymphangioma circumscriptum
K Molluscum contagiosum
L Neurofibroma
M Pyogenic granuloma
N Sebaceous cyst
O Seborrhoeic keratosis

The following scenarios describe patients presenting with benign cutaneous lesions. From the above list choose the most likely diagnosis. Each item may be used once, more than once, or not at all.

☐ **1** A 45-year-old carpenter presents with a lump over the dorsum of his right wrist that disappears on extension of the joint. The overlying skin is normal.

☐ **2** A 65-year-old woman presents with a lesion on her cheek that had rapidly increased in size over the last 6 weeks but has recently begun to get smaller. On examination she has a 9-mm hemispherical nodule that has a rolled edge and a central horny plug. There is no local lymphadenopathy.

☐ **3** A 3-year-old child attends after her parents notice a cluster of coloured small lumps in her axilla. She is otherwise well and her vaccinations are up to date. On examination there are multiple circumscribed 2–3-mm cystic-looking papules. Some are translucent while others are brown, red, or black in colour. These do not blanch with pressure.

☐ **4** A 35-year-old woman presents with a lump on her lower lip which has appeared rapidly over the last 6 days following a minor injury to the area. On examination there is a pink hemispherical nodule, 6 mm in diameter, that appears vascular and friable. There is no local lymphadenopathy.

108 THEME: PIGMENTED LESIONS OF THE SKIN

A Acral melanoma
B Amelanotic melanoma
C Blue naevus
D Café-au-lait patch
E Campbell de Morgan spot
F Compound naevus
G Deep capillary naevus
H Halo naevus
I Intradermal naevus
J Junctional naevus
K Lentigo
L Lentigo maligna (Hutchinson's malignant freckle)
M Mongolian blue spot
N Nodular melanoma
O Strawberry naevus
P Superficial capillary naevus
Q Superficial spreading melanoma

The following scenarios describe presentations of various pigmented lesions. From the above list choose the most appropriate diagnosis. Each item may be used once, more than once, or not at all.

☐ **1** A 6-year-old boy is brought in to clinic by his parents with a deep purple lesion over his right zygoma. It has been present since birth and he is otherwise well. On examination it extends over the entire cheek and is lumpy and thickened on palpation. There is no associated lymphadenopathy.

☐ **2** A 3-month-old baby is brought in by concerned parents who have noticed that a red lesion over his forehead, present from birth, has begun to reduce in size but has developed a black area centrally. There is no other lymphadenopathy and the child is otherwise developing normally.

☐ **3** A 35-year-old man presents with rectal bleeding and is noted to have multiple pigmented, small, flat moles around his mouth, on his lips and in the buccal membrane.

☐ **4** A 65-year-old woman presents with a rapidly growing, itchy, variegated, pigmented lesion on her arm. On examination there is a single flat black-brown area measuring 3 cm with an irregular margin surrounded by multiple smaller brown lesions.

109 THEME: MALIGNANT MELANOMA

A N_1 classification
B Stage III disease
C Stage IV disease
D T_1 lesion
E T_{2a} lesion
F T_{2b} lesion
G T_4 lesion

The following are descriptions which refer to malignant melanoma staging. Please select the most appropriate answer from the list above. The items may be used once, more than once, or not at all.

☐ **1** A 33-year-old woman has been referred with a possible diagnosis of cutaneous melanoma. On examination she has nodular malignant melanoma over the anterior aspect of her left leg. The lesion appears ulcerated. An excision biopsy is performed, the histology of which confirms an ulcerated, nodular malignant melanoma, Breslow's thickness of 1.79 mm. The lesion has been completely excised.

☐ **2** A 56-year-old man has presented with a hard fixed mass in his neck. On examination he is noted to have a superficial spreading melanoma on his forehead and, in addition, has multiple enlarged cervical lymph nodes. The rest of the examination is unremarkable. A fine-needle aspiration of the lymph nodes is performed along with an excision biopsy of the lymph nodes, the results of which confirm a superficial spreading malignant melanoma, Breslow's thickness of 2.32 mm. Cytology from the fine-needle aspirate reveals the presence of lymph node metastases. Subsequent staging scans reveal no evidence of distant metastases.

☐ **3** A 65-year-old woman is seen with a 1-month history of slowly progressive jaundice and weight loss. She also gives a 1-year history of nodule behind her right knee, which has recently started to ulcerate. She initially thought this was a cyst. On examination she is obviously icteric and appears wasted. Of note she is considerably short of breath at rest. Examination of her legs reveals an ulcerated nodular melanoma behind her right knee along with several enlarged inguinal lymph nodes on the same side. A hard irregular liver edge is found on palpation of her abdomen.

110 THEME: SKIN ULCERS

A Anthrax
B Basal cell carcinoma
C Chancrous ulcer
D Gummatous ulcer
E Ischaemic ulcer
F Marjolin's ulcer
G Mixed arteriovenous ulcer
H Neuropathic ulcer
I Pyoderma gangrenosum
J Squamous cell carcinoma
K Tuberculous ulcer
L Ulcerated melanoma
M Venous ulcer

The following are descriptions of patients with ulcers. Please select the most appropriate diagnosis from the list. The items may be used once, more than once, or not at all.

☐ **1** A 25-year-old man presents with a shallow, painless, round ulcer on his penis. On direct questioning he admits to having had unprotected sexual intercourse 1 month ago. The ulcer has a hard, raised, hyperaemic edge and there is associated shotty inguinal lymphadenopathy.

☐ **2** A 45-year-old farmer presents with septicaemia to The Emergency Department. A small ulcer with a black base and indurated edge is noticed on his forearm and there is axillary lymphadenopathy. He describes the ulcer starting as a small papule, which then broke down to form the ulcer.

Neurosurgery

111 THEME: HEAD INJURY (TYPES)

A	Basal skull fracture	G	Le Fort I fracture
B	Depressed skull fracture	H	Le Fort II fracture
C	Diffuse axonal injury	I	Le Fort III fracture
D	Extradural haematoma	J	Linear vault fracture
E	Intracerebral haemorrhage	K	Subarachnoid haemorrhage
F	Intraventricular haemorrhage	L	Subdural haematoma

The following patients have all sustained head injuries. Please select the most appropriate clinical description from the above list. The items may be used once, more than once, or not at all.

☐ **1** A 26-year-old man is assaulted with a baseball bat. On examination, he has multiple lacerations and bruises on his face. There is blood in the left external auditory meatus and bilateral black eyes with a left subconjunctival haematoma. Glasgow Coma Scale (GCS) is 15.

☐ **2** A 36-year-old unrestrained driver of a car is thrown against the dashboard and sustains facial injuries with significant haematomatous swelling over both maxillae and a flattening of the face. A skull X-ray and subsequent computed tomography (CT) reconstruction demonstrate a fracture extending from the nasal bridge below the nasofrontal suture through the frontal processes of the maxilla, inferolaterally through the lacrimal bones and inferior orbital floor and rim through the inferior orbital foramen, and inferiorly through the anterior wall of the maxillary sinus; it then travels under the zygoma, across the pterygomaxillary fissure, and through the pterygoid plates.

☐ **3** A 31-year-old falls from a height sustaining multiple injuries, including blunt injury to the head. She is deeply unconscious on arrival at The Emergency Department (GCS 3) with normal pupils. A CT scan demonstrates no focal abnormality but there is poor grey–white differentiation and loss of sulcal pattern with effacement of both lateral ventricles. The neurosurgeons place a monitoring bolt which demonstrates an intracranial pressure of 50 mmHG.

☐ **4** A 29-year-old woman with a history of epilepsy has a witnessed fit and fall with a blunt injury to the left side of her head with laceration. She recovers rapidly from the fit to a GCS of 15 by the time of her arrival in The Emergency Department and is awaiting a skull X-ray when she starts to become drowsy and confused. She is moved to the resuscitation area where her GCS declines rapidly to 7, requiring intubation.

112 THEME: HEAD INJURY (GLASGOW COMA SCALE; GCS)

A GCS 4
B GCS 5
C GCS 6
D GCS 7
E GCS 8
F GCS 9
G GCS 10
H GCS 11
I GCS 12
J GCS 13
K GCS 14

The following neurological observations are presented. Please select the appropriate score from the above list. The items may be used once, more than once, or not at all.

☐ **1** Eye opening; abnormal flexion to pain; best verbal response is 'incomprehensible sounds'.

☐ **2** Eye opening to speech; localises pain; best verbal response is 'confused conversation'.

☐ **3** Eye opening; normal flexion (withdrawal) to pain; best verbal response is 'inappropriate words'.

113 THEME: MANAGEMENT OPTIONS IN A PATIENT WITH HEAD INJURY

A Admit for neuro-observations
B Craniotomy
C Computed tomography (CT) scan
D Discharge
E Discharge and head injury instructions
F Elective burr hole
G Emergency burr hole
H Emergency laparotomy
I Endotracheal intubation
J Intracranial pressure monitoring
K Mannitol
L Mannitol and transfer to Neurosurgical Unit
M Skull X-ray

The following patients have all sustained head injuries. From the list above, select the most appropriate plan of management. The items may be used once, more than once, or not at all.

☐ **1** A 70-year-old woman attends The Emergency Department having fallen at home. She is unclear of the events surrounding the fall, and as she lives alone, no collateral history is available. She has vomited three times since arrival in the department. Her Glasgow Coma Scale (GCS) is currently 15. All other observations are normal. There is no evidence of focal neurological deficit.

☐ **2** A 24-year-old gentleman presents to The Emergency Department with a history of head injury while playing rugby. He was involved with a 'clash of heads' with another player during a 'ruck'. He remembers the events surrounding the event well, and has no amnesia. Collateral history from his friends confirms that there was no loss of consciousness. On examination he is fully orientated, GCS is 15 and all other observations are normal. There is no evidence of focal neurological deficit.

☐ **3** A 38-year-old gentleman has been involved in a road traffic accident and brought to The Emergency Department as a 'trauma call'. The ambulance staff inform you that he was a pedestrian hit by a car travelling at approximately 40 mph. He has sustained a significant head injury but the paramedic crew report that he was alert at the scene and that his pupils were equal and reactive. Having completed the primary survey, your examination reveals a GCS of 8, and a fixed dilated left pupil. There is no evidence of hemiparesis. No other significant injuries are apparent, and the patient is stable, and has a pulse rate of 50/min and a blood pressure of 160/80 mmHg. You request an urgent CT scan, but are informed that this will not be possible in your unit as the scanner is undergoing repair.

114 THEME: SPINAL CORD INJURY

A Anterior cord syndrome
B Brown–Sequard syndrome
C Central cord syndrome
D Complete spinal cord injury
E Conus lesion
F Incomplete spinal injury
G Neurogenic shock
H Spinal shock

The following patients have all sustained trauma, with involvement of the spinal cord. From the list above, select the most likely diagnosis. The items may be used once, more than once, or not at all.

☐ **1** A 22-year-old motorcyclist is involved in a road traffic accident with a car. On arrival in The Emergency Department he complains of severe pain between the shoulder blades, and of being 'unable to move his legs'. Primary survey reveals that he is able to maintain his own airway, and is breathing spontaneously. His pulse rate is 50/min, and his blood pressure is 90/50 mmHg. There are no signs of significant haemorrhage. Secondary survey and detailed neurological examination are deferred pending resuscitation, and stabilisation of vital signs.

☐ **2** An 18-year-old man falls from a height. There is no evidence of head injury. The primary survey is completed and all vital signs are normal and stable. Neurological examination reveals no sensory or motor function below the level of T8. Digital rectal examination is uncomfortable, and reveals normal voluntary contraction of the external anal sphincter.

☐ **3** A 78-year-old woman is found at the bottom of a flight of stairs. On arrival in The Emergency Department, the primary survey is completed, and neurological examination reveals loss of motor power in the upper limbs, and some mild weakness in the lower limbs. In addition, there is some sensory loss affecting the cervical dermatomes.

Trauma/orthopaedic surgery

115 THEME: COMPLICATIONS OF FRACTURES

A Associated injury: nerve
B Associated injury: vascular
C Associated injury: visceral
D Avascular necrosis (AVN)
E Compartment syndrome
F Complex regional pain syndrome (Sudeck's atrophy)
G Crush syndrome
H Deep venous thrombosis
I Delayed union
J Fat embolism
K Hypovolaemic shock
L Malunion
M Myositis ossificans
N Non-union
O Osteomyelitis
P Pulmonary embolus

The above list documents complications of fractures. Please pick the most appropriate complication for the following clinical scenarios. Each item may be used once, more than once, or not at all.

☐ **1** A 35-year-old footballer has been admitted to the ward having sustained a spiral fracture to his right tibia. He is awaiting surgery and currently has a plaster backslab protecting his leg. The nurses on the ward have called you multiple times to ask for stronger analgesia, which apparently is still not settling his pain. When you assess him he is fidgeting in the bed. He complains of significant pain at the site of his fracture and some numbness between his great and second toe. He has warm, pink toes, and a dorsalis pedis pulse can just be palpated beneath the plaster and bandaging.

☐ **2** A 29-year-old woman who dislocated her left elbow 4 weeks ago, during a strenuous martial arts training session, is being followed up in fracture clinic. (The elbow had been successfully re-located in a closed manoeuvre in Casualty). She tells you that after an initially good recovery, movement of the joint has suddenly become restricted and very painful. On closer questioning you determine that she has been rather actively mobilising the joint from an early stage to attempt to get back to her martial arts. An X-ray shows some calcification anterior to the joint.

☐ **3** A 45-year-old woman, who fell from her horse 3 months ago, returns for follow-up in orthopaedic outpatients. At the time her notes documented a dorsiflexion injury to her left wrist causing a scaphoid fracture that was treated in a scaphoid cast for 8 weeks.

She continues to have pain and weakness in her left wrist despite a course of physiotherapy. The X-ray that you request shows increased density at the proximal pole of the scaphoid.

☐ **4** A 27-year-old rugby player presents to Casualty after being tackled to the ground during a match. His team-mates give an account of a forceful shoulder blow to his left chest. On examination he has significant bruising over his lower left chest and this region feels boggy. Clinically two ribs appear fractured. As you assess him further he starts to complain of severe shortness of breath and his breath sounds are diminished on the left side. Percussion note is hyper-resonant. SaO_2: 89% on air, respiratory rate 35 breaths/min.

116 THEME: COMMON FRACTURE EPONYMS

A Barton's fracture
B Bennett's fracture
C Colles' fracture
D Galeazzi's fracture dislocation
E Garden II fracture
F Garden III fracture
G Garden IV fracture
H Hill–Sachs fracture
I Lisfranc fracture dislocation
J Monteggia's fracture dislocation
K Rolando's fracture
L Smith's fracture
M Weber A fracture
N Weber B fracture
O Weber C fracture

The following are descriptions of fractures. Please select the most appropriate fracture eponym from the above list. Each item may be used once, more than once, or not at all. These are all commonly used in current clinical practice (and so remain important).

☐ **1** A comminuted, intra-articular fracture to the base of the first metacarpal.

☐ **2** A distal fibular fracture at the level of the syndesmosis, with or without a malleolar fracture.

☐ **3** A complete fracture through the femoral neck, with rotation of the femoral head within the acetabulum, demonstrating minimal displacement.

☐ **4** An intra-articular fracture of the volar or dorsal margin of the distal radius. The fracture extends obliquely to the radio-carpal joint with a striking dislocation of the carpus.

117 THEME: TREATMENT OPTIONS IN FRACTURE MANAGEMENT

A Broad arm sling (polysling)
B Cast-brace
C Cerclage wires
D Dynamic screw fixation
E External fixation
F Hanging cast
G Hemiarthroplasty
H Intramedullary nailing
I K-wires
J Plaster cast
K Plate and screw fixation
L Screw fixation
M Tension band wiring
N Traction

All of the above are employed in the management of fractures. For the following fractures please choose the most appropriate method of fracture fixation from the list. Each item may be used once, more than once, or not at all.

☐ **1** A closed, two-part fracture to the middle third of the clavicle (low-impact mechanism).

☐ **2** An inter-trochanteric fracture to the left neck of the femur in a 75-year-old woman.

☐ **3** An isolated femoral shaft fracture in a 4-year-old boy.

☐ **4** A Gustilo III comminuted tibial fracture in a 35-year-old man.

118 THEME: COMMON DISORDERS OF THE HAND

A Carpal tunnel syndrome
B Dupuytren's disease
C Extensor tendon injury
D Flexor tendon injury
E Gamekeeper's thumb
F Ganglion
G Heberden's node
H Mallet finger
I Paronychia
J Phalangeal endochondroma
K Pulp space infection
L Pyogenic granuloma
M Rheumatoid arthritis
N Trigger finger

The following patients present with disorders of the hand. From the list above, select the most likely diagnosis. The items may be used once, more than once, or not at all.

☐ **1** A 44-year-old man attends the clinic and reports that his index finger often gets stuck and 'clicks' when he straightens it. He denies any history of trauma. He has no relevant past medical history. On examination, the finger, and rest of the hand, appears normal. There is no contracture of the skin or subcutaneous tissues. Initially, the index finger is fixed in flexion, but it suddenly extends fully during active movement. There is no associated pain.

☐ **2** A 64-year-old woman attends The Emergency Department with a fracture of the distal phalanx of her left middle finger. She informs you that this finger has become increasingly painful over the last few months, and that she has been aware of a 'bony swelling' affecting this finger. She indicates that this was most marked on the volar aspect of the distal phalanx, close to the distal interphalangeal joint.

☐ **3** A 28-year-old manual labourer attends The Emergency Department with a painful left index finger. He sustained a minor abrasion to the palmar aspect of his left index finger at work 6 days ago. On examination, there is erythema and swelling affecting the distal aspect of the left index finger on the palmar surface.

119 THEME: MONO- AND POLYARTHRITIS

A	Behçet's syndrome	H	Rheumatoid arthritis
B	Drug allergies	I	Septic arthritis
C	Gout	J	Spondyloarthritides
D	Osteoarthritis	K	Still's disease
E	Pseudogout	L	Systemic lupus erythematosus
F	Psoriasis	M	Trauma
G	Reiter's syndrome	N	Viral illness

The following patients all present with symptoms of arthritis. From the list above, select the most likely diagnosis. The items may be used once, more than once, or not at all.

☐ **1** A 43-year-old man attends The Emergency Department with a painful right knee. He reports a sudden onset of severe, constant pain in the right knee, and that he is no longer able to mobilise. His temperature is 38.5 °C. Examination of the knee reveals an increased temperature over the right knee, but no erythema. He is tender in the joint line, and he is unable to actively move the joint.

☐ **2** A 52-year-old woman attends the clinic with a long history of intermittent pain and swelling affecting her left knee. Past history includes hypothyroidism. Examination is unremarkable. A plain radiograph reveals the presence of intra-articular calcium deposition, but no other abnormality.

☐ **3** A 13-year-old girl is referred with a 6-month history of pain and swelling affecting the joints of her upper limbs. Her mother also informs you that she also suffers with a 'grumbling appendix'. On examination, there is bilateral involvement of the shoulder joints, elbows and wrists. Abdominal examination reveals splenomegaly.

120 THEME: COMPLICATIONS OF RHEUMATOID ARTHRITIS

A Anaemia
B Boutonnière's deformity
C Bronchiolitis obliterans
D Carpal tunnel syndrome
E Felty's syndrome
F Joint subluxation
G Mononeuritis
H Ocular disease
I Pericarditis
J Peripheral neuropathy
K Pleural effusion
L Renal disease
M Rheumatoid nodules
N Swan neck deformity
O Thrombocytosis
P Vascular lesions
Q Z deformity of the thumb

Above is a list of potential complications of rheumatoid arthritis. For the following scenarios please pick the most appropriate complication. Each item may be used once, more than once, or not at all.

☐ **1** A 60-year-old woman presents with worsening deformity of her hands. On examination you note flexion at the proximal interphalangeal joint of the middle finger on her left hand, with hyperextension at the distal interphalangeal joint. Her metacarpophalangeal joint is extended.

☐ **2** A 64-year-old gentleman with a chronic history of rheumatoid arthritis presents to the elderly day ward with a history of malaise and lethargy. On examination he has splenomegaly with generalised lymphadenopathy; you also notice some weeping leg ulcers. A full blood count shows a pancytopenia (white cell count 2.4×10^9/litre, haemoglobin 10.5 g/dl, platelets 95×10^9/litre).

☐ **3** A 50-year-old man presents to The Emergency Department complaining of a progressive shortness of breath. Previously fit and well, he now describes dyspnoea on mild exertion. On examination he has decreased breath sounds at the left lung base and this region is dull to percussion.

☐ **4** A 48-year-old woman with known rheumatoid arthritis presents to outpatients complaining of pain and paraesthesia to her thumb, forefinger and middle finger of her right hand. The symptoms have been progressive and are worse at night. In clinic you are able to reproduce her symptoms using Phalen's test.

121 THEME: UPPER LIMB INJURIES

A Anterior dislocation of the shoulder
B Acromioclavicular joint dislocation
C Colles' fracture
D Fracture of the clavicle
E Fracture dislocation of the elbow
F Fracture of the distal humerus
G Fracture of the proximal humerus
H Fracture of the radial head
I Fractured scapula
J Fractured shaft of humerus
K Olecranon fracture
L Posterior dislocation of the shoulder
M Scaphoid fracture
N Smith's fracture
O Sternoclavicular dislocation
P Supracondylar fracture of the humerus

The following patients have all fallen, injuring their upper limb. Please select the most appropriate fracture or dislocation from the above list. The items may be used once, more than once, or not at all.

☐ **1** A 20-year-old epileptic presents to The Emergency Department following a seizure. On recovering from his seizure he complains of pain in his right arm. In addition, he is unable to move the affected limb. On examination his right arm is medially rotated at the shoulder. Active and passive movement is not possible at the shoulder joint. There is no obvious neurovascular deficit.

☐ **2** A 60-year-old woman has fallen onto her outstretched hand. On presentation she has marked bruising and tenderness of the upper arm. Neurovascular examination reveals wrist drop.

☐ **3** A 24-year-old man presents after falling onto his outstretched hand. He complains of pain at the elbow. Examination reveals swelling around the elbow. Of note, the patient is unable to extend the elbow against resistance. There is no obvious neurovascular deficit.

122 THEME: BACK PAIN

A	Ankylosing spondylitis	G	Scheuermann's disease
B	Intervertebral disc herniation	H	Spinal stenosis
C	Metastatic carcinoma	I	Spinal trauma
D	Mutiple myeloma	J	Spondylolisthesis
E	Osteoporosis	K	Spondylosis
F	Osteomyelitis	L	Tuberculosis

From the list above, select the most likely diagnosis for the following patients who all present with back pain. The items may be used once, more than once, or not at all.

☐ **1** A 73-year-old diabetic man complains of severe back pain following an anterior resection. On examination, his temperature is 38.1 °C, there is a limited range of spinal movements and marked lumbar muscle spasm. Neurological examination is normal.

☐ **2** A 57-year-old woman presents to The Emergency Department with progressive severe thoracic back pain that has not responded to simple analgesics. The pain is now constant, and interrupts her sleep.

☐ **3** A 65-year-old woman is referred for assessment of chronic lower back pain. Past history includes rheumatoid arthritis, for which she uses long-term steroids. She underwent a total abdominal hysterectomy and bilateral salpingo-oophorectomy at the age of 35 years. There is no neurological deficit on examination.

123 THEME: BONE AND SOFT TISSUE TUMOURS

A Bone metastases
B Chondroma
C Chondrosarcoma
D Ewing's sarcoma
E Fibroma
F Fibrosarcoma
G Leiomyoma
H Leiomyosarcoma
I Lipoma
J Liposarcoma
K Osteoma
L Osteoblastoma
M Osteochondroma
N Osteosarcoma (osteogenic sarcoma)
O Osteoid osteoma
P Simple bone cyst

The following patients all present with bone or soft tissue tumours. From the list above, select the most likely diagnosis. The items may be used once, more than once, or not at all.

☐ **1** A 15-year-old boy attends The Emergency Department. He describes pain affecting his left femur that was initially an ache but that has now become severe and constant. In addition, he reports generalised malaise and a persistent cough. On examination, he has an antalgic gait and there is asymmetrical swelling affecting the distal left femur. Radiology reveals breach of the periosteum, which is elevated, and a 'sunray' appearance affecting the distal femur.

☐ **2** A 51-year-old woman is referred urgently by her general practitioner with 'a right upper quadrant mass, which he suspects is malignant'. On examination, there is no evidence of an abdominal mass but there is a tender swelling arising from the right costal margin. An X-ray of the lesion reveals a localised area of bone destruction with mottled appearances, affecting the ninth rib near the costal margin.

☐ **3** A 12-year-old girl is referred with pain and swelling affecting her left lower leg. On examination, there is a tender, irregular swelling arising from the mid-tibia. X-ray reveals a destructive lesion, associated with a soft tissue mass, and peri-osteal 'onion-skinning'. Biopsy demonstrates the presence of sheets of 'small round cells'.

124 THEME: PAINFUL CONDITIONS OF THE FOOT

A Claw toe
B Freiberg's disease
C Gout
D Hallux rigidus
E Hallux valgus
F Hammer toe
G March fracture
H Morton's metatarsalgia
I Pes cavus
J Rheumatoid arthritis
K Sever's disease

The following descriptions are of patients who have presented with painful conditions of the foot. Please select the most appropriate diagnosis from the above list. The items may be used once, more than once, or not at all.

☐ **1** A 45-year-old woman presents with a history of a sharp pain over the dorsum of the foot, which radiates into her toes. Examination reveals a fine point of tenderness in the cleft between the third and fourth toes.

☐ **2** A 25-year-old nurse asks for your opinion regarding her painful left foot. She qualified 5 months ago and has been working in The Emergency Department since. The pain started 1 week ago and causes her to limp. On examination she is tender over the second metatarsal, which feels unusually thick.

☐ **3** A 42-year-old man complains of sudden onset of pain over the medial aspect of his right forefoot. Of note, he has recently returned from a 'stag' weekend in Dublin. On examination the base of his big toe is swollen, erythematous, hot and tender to touch.

☐ **4** A 23-year-old woman presents with a history of pain in the sole of her foot and on the dorsal aspect of her second toe. On examination there are callosities over the proximal interphalangeal joint of the second toe, which appears flexed and under the second metatarsal head. The second metatarsophalangeal and distal interphalangeal joints appear hyperextended.

☐ **5** A 10 year-old boy presents with pain in his right heel. On examination, the foot appears grossly normal, however there is significant tenderness over the calcaneum close to the insertion of the Achilles tendon.

125 THEME: THE PAINFUL KNEE

- A Anterior cruciate injury
- B Chondromalacia patellae
- C Infrapatellar bursitis
- D Lateral collateral injury
- E Medial collateral injury
- F Meniscal tear
- G Osgood–Schlatter disease
- H Osteoarthritis
- I Osteochondritis dessicans
- J Pre-patellar bursitis
- K Recurrent dislocation of the patella
- L Rheumatoid arthritis
- M Septic arthritis
- N Tendinitis

The following are descriptions of patients with a painful knee(s). Please select the most appropriate diagnosis from the above list. The items may be used once, more than once, or not at all.

☐ **1** A 43-year-old woman is seen with a history of chronic pain and swelling of the knee. On examination, flexion and extension of the knee are limited and a marked valgus deformity is noted. This is particularly apparent on standing.

☐ **2** A 14-year-old girl is seen with a 3-month history of knee pain. There is no history of trauma. The pain is felt principally in front of the knee and is exacerbated on ascending and descending stairs.

☐ **3** A 19-year-old man presents with a history of intermittent pain and swelling in his left knee. In addition, he complains of his knee locking, which he relieves by manoeuvring the leg. He also complains of his knee 'giving way.' There is no history of trauma. On examination a small effusion is noted and a small mobile 'body' is felt in the suprapatellar pouch.

126 THEME: KNEE INJURIES

A Anterior cruciate ligament (ACL) injury
B Extensor mechanism disruption
C Knee dislocation
D Lateral collateral ligament injury
E Medial collateral ligament injury
F Meniscal tear
G Neck of fibular fracture
H Patellar dislocation
I Patellar fracture
J Posterior cruciate ligament (PCL) injury
K Proximal tibio-fibular dislocation
L Supracondylar fracture
M Tibial plateau fracture

The above are all descriptions of injuries to the knee. For the following scenarios please select the most appropriate answer from the list. The items may be used once, more than once, or not at all.

☐ **1** A 30-year-old footballer, playing in the Sunday league, presents to The Emergency Department minors on Monday evening. He is complaining of a swollen right knee with pain, and an inability to completely straighten the joint. He describes the injury occurring as he tried to break into a run on the muddy pitch. His right thigh twisted but his leg remained fixed in the mud. At the time, although his knee was painful, he had not noticed any swelling and had continued to play. This morning he had observed that his right knee was much larger in size than the other. He has tenderness along the lateral joint line.

☐ **2** A 60-year-old grandfather presents acutely to the Casualty department complaining of severe pain in his left knee. He tells you that he was playing with his grandson who had unexpectedly jumped up on him from behind, causing him to stumble and lunge forward. As he lurched forward he noticed a sudden searing pain in his thigh and knee and was immediately unable to walk on the affected leg. On examination he is holding his knee in slight flexion and is unable to fully straighten the joint. He is incapable of performing a straight leg raise. An X-ray does not reveal any fracture.

☐ **3** A 35-year-old skier has been flown back to the UK from the Alps after injuring himself on the slopes. He describes a 'twisting' injury to his left knee as his ski caught in some soft snow. Immediately he felt an agonising pain, heard a 'pop' and noticed instantaneous swelling, under his salopettes. He was unable to carry on skiing and after hobbling down the piste was seen by the resort doctor who has documented a positive Lachman test.

☐ **4** A 28-year-old woman is brought into Casualty by ambulance following an accident while parachuting with the Territorial Army. She landed badly and forcefully on her left knee, which was flexed at the time. She complains of pain and tingling on the dorsum of her foot, and she cannot dorsiflex at the left ankle. X-ray of the knee does not clearly show any fracture.

127 THEME: THE CHILDHOOD LIMP

A Acquired dislocation of the hip
B Congenital dislocation of the hip
C Congenital subluxation
D Non-specific transient tenosynovitis
E Perthes' disease
F Pyogenic arthritis
G Slipped upper femoral epiphysis
H Still's disease
I Tuberculous synovitis

The following are descriptions of children who have presented with a limp. Please select the most appropriate diagnosis from the above list. The items may be used once, more than once, or not at all.

☐ **1** A 14-year-old boy is brought to The Emergency Department by his mother. She is worried as he fell 4 days ago and has continued to limp since. He gives a 6-month history of pain in his right knee, which has worsened since falling over. On examination he is considerably overweight and has evidence of delayed puberty. His right leg is externally rotated and appears to be shorter than the left. Assessment of limb movements is not possible because of excessive pain in the limb.

☐ **2** A 7-year-old boy is seen in clinic with a history of a limp and pain in the left groin. Initially the pain was severe and he was unable to move his left leg. The pain resolved spontaneously after bed rest. One month later his symptoms have now recurred with a similar, less severe pain, which causes him to limp. Examination of the left lower limb is normal except for limited abduction and internal rotation of the left hip.

☐ **3** A 7-year-old girl is seen in the paediatric Emergency Department with a 1-day history of sudden onset of pain in the left hip and difficulty in ambulation. On examination she is apyrexial, appears well and is lying with her hip flexed and externally rotated. Palpation of her hip reveals tenderness over the anterior aspect. Extension, abduction and internal rotation lead to severe pain. Initial investigations include a full blood count, erythrocyte sedimentation rate and plain radiographs, all of which are normal.

☐ **4** A 5-year-old girl is seen with a history of a limp. Her father says that she has been unwell recently with an intermittent fever. On examination she has an obvious limp when walking and is pyrexial (temperature 37.9 °C). Examination reveals mild tenderness over the right hip, with a generalised reduction in movement. Her erythrocyte sedimentation rate is raised and her serum is positive for antinuclear antibodies.

Urology

128 THEME: HAEMATURIA

A	Acute prostatitis	I	Prostatic adenocarcinoma
B	Anticoagulation therapy	J	Pyelonephritis
C	Benign prostatic hyperplasia	K	Renal cell carcinoma
D	Bladder cancer	L	Renal papillary necrosis
E	Cystitis	M	Trauma
F	Haemophilia	N	Urethral caruncle
G	Nephritis	O	Urethritis
H	Polycystic kidney disease	P	Urolithiasis

The following patients all present with haematuria. From the list above, select the most likely diagnosis. The items may be used once, more than once, or not at all.

☐ **1** A 32-year-old man attends The Emergency Department with frank haematuria. He describes a several month history of bilateral loin pain, followed by the recent onset of frank haematuria. On examination, his blood pressure is 165/100 mmHg and he is tender in both renal angles. Abdominal examination reveals bilateral lumbar abdominal masses. Urinalysis: 3+ blood and protein. Urea & Electrolytes: Na^+ 138 mmol/litre, K^+ 5.6 mmol/litre, urea 13.6 mmol/litre, creatinine 195 μmol/litre.

☐ **2** A 56-year-old diabetic woman presents to The Emergency Department with severe colicky right loin pain followed by the passage of blood-stained material per urethrum with subsequent resolution of the pain. She currently takes non-steroidal anti-inflammatory agents for chronic back pain. Urinalysis reveals microscopic haematuria. A kidney and upper bladder X-ray demonstrates ring-shaped calcification, in the distribution of both kidneys. An intravenous urogram film obtained at 5 min shows horns from the calices and ring shadows. There are no other obvious filling defects.

☐ **3** A 75-year-old woman is referred with painless microscopic haematuria. She has also noticed a bloody discharge staining her underwear. On examination, there are no abdominal masses, inspection of the perineum reveals a red mass at the urethral meatus. Intravenous urogram and cystoscopy are normal.

129 THEME: INVESTIGATION OF URINARY TRACT DISORDERS

A Antegrade ureteropyelography
B Computed tomography (CT)
C Computed tomography urography (CTU)
D Cystourethroscopy
E DMSA (dimercaptosuccinic acid) scan
F Intravenous ureterogram (IVU)
G Kidney, ureter and bladder (KUB) X-ray
H MAG 3 scan
I Magnetic resonance imaging (MRI)
J Renal angiography
K Retrograde ureteropyelography
L Transrectal prostatic biopsy
M Transrectal ultrasound (TRUS)
N Ultrasound kidneys, ureters and bladder
O Urethrography and cystography
P Urodynamic studies

The above are all examples of investigations used in the diagnosis of urinary tract disorders. Please pick the most appropriate investigation for the following clinical presentations/descriptions. The items may be used once, more than once, or not at all.

☐ **1** A 62-year-old man presents to The Emergency Department complaining of haematuria, gnawing right loin pain and malaise. Abdominal examination does not reveal anything grossly abnormal. Urine cytology and culture are normal. An ultrasound is performed urgently and shows a complex right renal cyst with a calcified wall and a more solid central component. The patient tells you that he has had a prior allergic reaction to an injected contrast that he had in his 50s for some form of abdominal investigation. How should he be further investigated?

☐ **2** A 40-year-old woman who is an inpatient on the Urology Ward recently had a left-sided percutaneous nephrostomy tube sited for pyonephrosis. This was performed as an emergency procedure on her admission with sepsis and right loin pain, following an ultrasound KUB showing left-sided hydronephrosis. Urea 15 mmol/litre; creatinine 205 µmol/litre. What further imaging should be undertaken to assess the cause of her infected kidney?

☐ **3** A 50-year-old smoker presents to the urology outpatients after referral by his general practitioner for painless haematuria. His prostate feels smooth and of normal size and he denies any lower urinary tract symptoms. All relevant blood tests and urine samples have been taken and show nothing of significance other than confirming haematuria. You need to arrange the next investigation.

130 THEME: BLADDER OUTFLOW OBSTRUCTION

A Benign prostatic hyperplasia (BPH)
B Bladder neck dyssynergia
C Bladder neck stone
D Bladder neck tumour
E Carcinoma of the prostate
F Clot retention
G Detrusor-external sphincter dyssynergia (DESD)
H Neuropathic bladder
I Pelvic mass/tumour
J Pelvic organ prolapse
K Previous bladder neck suspension surgery
L Urethral diverticulae
M Urethral dysfunction
N Urethral stone
O Urethral stricture

The pathologies above can all contribute to bladder outflow obstruction. For the following scenarios please pick the most appropriate cause from the list. The items may be used once, more than once, or not at all.

☐ **1** A 52-year-old man presents to the urology outpatient department complaining of a progressively 'poor stream' over the past few weeks. He tells you that he was recently an in-patient, having undergone coronary artery bypass graft surgery, and that he required an in-dwelling catheter for 6 weeks after suffering complications from the surgery post-operatively. Before this he had had no urinary symptoms at all.

☐ **2** A 73-year-old man finally presents to his general practitioner (GP) after an 18-month history of urinary symptoms. He was previously too embarrassed to discuss his worsening hesitancy, post-micturition dribbling and nocturia. You later see him in the outpatients on his GP's referral. On examination his abdomen is unremarkable and his prostate appears smoothly enlarged. Prostate-specific antigen 5.0 ng/ml.

☐ **3** A 58-year-old man presents to The Emergency Department complaining of severe suprapubic pain and an inability to pass urine for the preceding 12 h. He tells you that he was recently discharged from hospital following a transurethral resection of bladder tumour procedure.

☐ **4** A 35-year-old professional show jumper who had sustained a spinal cord injury after a fall from his horse 1 month prior, is seen in the urology outpatients. On leaving hospital after his initial injury he was reluctant to have a long-term urinary catheter and it was agreed that he should try intermittent self-catheterisation (ISC) under the supervision of the community continence nurse. He admits to you that he has been a little unenthusiastic with the catheterisation in the past week (only emptying once or twice a day) and had been experiencing some leaking in between attempts. On examination he has a distended bladder. On siting a catheter, approximately 800 ml of clear urine drains rapidly. A voiding cystourethrogram shows a voluminous bladder and every time the patient tries to pass urine a narrowing is observed in the urethra between the prostatic and bulbar urethra. Urea 16 mmol/litre; creatinine 240 µmol/litre.

131 THEME: DISORDERS OF THE PROSTATE

A Acute prostatitis
B Benign prostatic hyperplasia
C Carcinoma of the prostate
D Chronic prostatitis
E Granulomatous prostatitis
F Prostatic abscess
G Prostatodynia

From the list above, select the most likely diagnosis for the following patients with disorders of the prostate. The items may be used once, more than once, or not at all.

☐ **1** A 72-year-old diabetic gentleman is referred for assessment of lower urinary tract symptoms. He reports worsening frequency of micturition and nocturia. He has also noticed difficulties initiating micturition, and terminal dribbling. Abdominal examination is normal, digital examination per rectum reveals a non-tender, enlarged prostate gland. Urinalysis reveals microscopic haematuria. The following investigation results are available: haemoglobin 13.4 g/dl, white cell count 5.4×10^9/litre, platelets 254×10^9/litre, Na^+ 132 mmol/litre, K^+ 5.3 mmol/litre, urea 9.8 mmol/litre, creatinine 165 µmol/litre, prostate-specific antigen 4.2 ng/ml.

☐ **2** A 34-year-old gentleman presents to The Emergency Department with acute retention of urine. He reports worsening dysuria over the last few days, associated with rigors and night sweats. He is currently taking triple immunosuppression therapy following heart and lung transplantation for cystic fibrosis. Vital observations: temperature 38.9 °C, pulse rate 125/min, blood pressure 90/46 mmHg, respiratory rate 16 breaths/min, SaO_2 98%. Digital per rectal examination reveals a tender boggy prostate that is fluctuant.

☐ **3** A 65-year-old gentleman presents with a history of abdominal distension and pain, and worsening constipation. On direct questioning he also reports marked perineal pain. Urinalysis reveals microscopic haematuria. Urea & Electrolytes reveal evidence of renal failure: Na^+ 132 mmol/litre, K^+ 5.9 mmol/litre, urea 20.6 mmol/litre, creatinine 256 µmol/litre.

132 THEME: URINARY INCONTINENCE

A Acute retention of urine
B Chronic retention of urine
C Detrusor overactivity
D Detrusor hypotonia
E Faecal impaction
F Fistulation
G Functional
H Urethral diverticulum
I Urethral sphincter incompetence
J Urethral stricture
K Urinary tract infection
L Uterovaginal prolapse

The following patients all present with urinary incontinence. From the list above, select the most likely diagnosis. The items may be used once, more than once, or not at all.

☐ **1** A 68-year-old woman complains of worsening urinary incontinence. She reports loss of a trickle of urine when coughing or during physical exertion. She denies urinary frequency and urgency. In the past she has had four normal vaginal deliveries. Urine culture is normal. On examination, there is no evidence of urinary retention clinically, vaginal examination excludes significant prolapse. There is objective loss of urine on coughing.

☐ **2** A 72-year-old man presents with symptoms of urinary incontinence. The loss is associated with marked urinary urgency and is worse when the 'weather is cold'. He has a 15-year history of bladder outflow obstruction. He recently underwent transurethral resection of the prostate, which has been associated with a deterioration of his continence.

☐ **3** A 48-year-old woman complains of 'constantly being wet – day and night' following a radical hysterectomy and radiotherapy for cervical cancer. Urinalysis and urodynamic investigations are normal.

133 THEME: SCROTAL SWELLINGS

A Acute epididymo-orchitis
B Acute haematocoele
C Chronic haematocoele
D Epididymal cyst
E Inguinal hernia
F Orchitis
G Primary hydrocoele
H Secondary hydrocoele
I Testicular seminoma
J Testicular teratoma
K Testicular torsion
L Tuberculous epididymo-orchitis
M Varicocoele

The above are all potential causes of a swelling in the scrotum. For the ensuing clinical scenarios please pick the most appropriate answer from the list. Each item may be used once, more than once, or not at all.

☐ **1** A 16-year-old presents to his general practitioner (GP) complaining of a vague, dragging sensation and aching in the left scrotum. The GP examines him lying flat and cannot identify anything unremarkable within either hemi-scrotum. On standing, however, there is a soft area of bulging swelling that appears in the left upper scrotum.

☐ **2** A 13-year-old boy presents to Casualty in the early hours of the morning complaining of unbearable pain in his left scrotum. The onset was sudden, woke him from sleep and caused him to vomit.

☐ **3** A 47-year-old man presents to the urology outpatient clinic with a 3–4-year history of a slowly enlarging, non-tender swelling in his right scrotum. On examination you note a multilocular 2-cm swelling located at the upper, posterior pole of the right testis. It is fluctuant, transmits a fluid thrill and transilluminates. The cord is easily palpated above the bulge.

☐ **4** A 27-year-old man attends The Emergency Department complaining of bilateral testicular pain and swelling. He gives a 5-day history of fever and malaise and tells you that he had some bilateral jaw swelling and pain that appears to be settling now. On examination he has a temperature of 38.9 °C; his testes are swollen, tender to palpation and feel somewhat soft.

134 THEME: HEMISCROTAL PAIN

A Acute epididymo-orchitis
B Chronic post-vasectomy pain
C Fournier's gangrene
D Hydrocoele
E Inguinoscrotal hernia
F Orchitis
G Referred pain
H Testicular injury
I Testicular torsion
J Testicular tumour
K Tuberculous epidydimo-orchitis
L Torsion of testicular appendage
M Varicocoele

The following patients all present with hemiscrotal pain. From the list above, select the most likely diagnosis. The items may be used once, more than once, or not at all.

☐ **1** A 9-year-old boy attends The Emergency Department with a sudden onset of severe pain in the left hemiscrotum, which is associated with lower abdominal discomfort. There is no history of trauma. He is in pain but afebrile. Examination of the external genitalia reveals normal position of both testicles, and no erythema or increased temperature. The left testicle is exquisitely tender over a small area on the upper pole, and there is marked thickening of the cord.

☐ **2** A 58-year-old diabetic gentleman develops worsening scrotal pain following drainage of a peri-anal abscess. He is unwell and has a temperature of 38.5 °C. Examination of his external genitalia reveals a painful, erythematous swollen right scrotum. The swelling also appears to be extending into the right inguinal region, and to a lesser degree, the left scrotum.

☐ **3** A 33-year-old man presents to The Emergency Department with a 7-day history of pain affecting the right hemiscrotum. On direct questioning, he reports symptoms of dysuria preceding the onset of the pain. There is no history of trauma. On examination, his temperature is 37.9 °C, and his right scrotum appears enlarged compared to the left. Palpation of scrotal contents reveals a tender thickening posterior to the testis, which itself is relatively painless.

135 THEME: RENAL MASSES

A Hydronephrosis
B Nephroblastoma (Wilm's tumour)
C Peri-nephric abscess
D Polycystic disease
E Renal cell carcinoma
F Renal haematoma
G Solitary cysts
H Supernumerary kidney

From the list above, select the most likely diagnosis for the following patients who all present with enlargement of the kidney on physical examination. The items may be used once, more than once, or not at all.

☐ **1** A 59-year-old man is found to have enlargement of his right kidney on physical examination. Past history includes emergency repair of a ruptured abdominal aortic aneurysm 5 years ago. Urinalysis is normal, and no malignant cells are seen on microscopy. His Urea & Electrolytes are normal.

☐ **2** A 4-year-old boy is referred by his general practitioner with an enlarged left kidney. He is otherwise asymptomatic and completely well. He is afebrile. Urinalysis reveals microscopic haematuria. Urine cultures are negative.

☐ **3** A 39-year-old woman is referred for assessment by an The Emergency Department Senior House Officer who has identified a tender right renal mass. She tells you that she has been unwell for several days, when she has been anorexic, suffering with night sweats and generalised malaise. Previously, she has noted frequency of micturition. There is no history of trauma. She presented to The Emergency Department with ureteric colic 5 days ago but was discharged because the pain appeared to settle. Urinalysis reveals 3+ of blood and protein.

136 THEME: TUMOURS OF THE GENITOURINARY TRACT

A Carcinoma of the penis
B Carcinoma of the urethra
C Cervical carcinoma
D Nephroblastoma (Wilm's tumour)
E Ovarian carcinoma
F Prostatic carcinoma
G Renal cell carcinoma
H Squamous cell carcinoma of the bladder
I Testicular cancer
J Transitional cell carcinoma of the bladder
K Transitional cell carcinoma of the ureter
L Uterine carcinoma
M Vaginal carcinoma
N Vulval carcinoma

The following patients all present with genitourinary tract malignancies. From the list above, select the most likely diagnosis. The items may be used once, more than once, or not at all.

☐ **1** A 54-year-old woman attends The Emergency Department with a 2-day history of frank haematuria. On direct questioning, she reports a several month history of irritative lower urinary tract symptoms. Her general practitioner has been treating her for recurrent urinary tract infections as urinalysis has repeatedly revealed the presence of microscopic haematuria. However, urine cultures have all been negative. She has noticed that the bleeding over the last few days only affects the end of her stream. She has smoked 40 per day for the last 40 years.

☐ **2** A 64-year-old nulliparous woman presents with increasing abdominal distension and pain. Previously, she was completely asymptomatic but more recently has also become increasingly short of breath. On examination, there is evidence of a left pleural effusion and gross ascites.

☐ **3** A 56-year-old man attends The Emergency Department with frank haematuria and some vague abdominal pain. On examination there is a swelling in the right loin.

ANSWERS

ANSWERS

PRINCIPLES OF SURGERY IN GENERAL

Peri-operative care

1 PRE-OPERATIVE FITNESS FOR SURGERY

This question tests your knowledge of the obligatory pre-operative investigations as stated in the NICE (National Institute for Clinical Excellence) guidelines. It should be noted that these are only guidelines and it is likely that your clinical practice and that of your anaesthetist may vary. You should however have a look at them.

1 I – No investigation required

Anyone between the ages of 16 and 39 years who is ASA (American Society of Anaesthesiologists) Grade 1 does not require any investigations prior to a minor procedure. The ASA grading system consists of five levels (1–5) and allows classification of a patient's co-morbidity with respect to anaesthetic risk. Grade 1 is associated with minimum risk and includes healthy normal patients, ie with no clinically important co-morbidity and without a clinically significant past/present medical history.

2 E – Full blood count (FBC), electrocardiogram and Urea & Electrolytes

These are the obligatory investigations for an ASA Grade 2 or Grade 3 patient with cardiovascular disease. Investigations that the NICE guidelines suggest should be *considered* include chest X-ray, urine analysis and blood gases.

3 E – FBC, electrocardiogram and Urea & Electrolytes

These three investigations are the minimum required for major and major, complex (Grade 3 and 4) types of surgery for most ASA grades 2 and 3. In this particular scenario, a chest X-ray, clotting studies, random glucose, blood gases and urine analysis should also be considered.

2 CONSENT FOR SURGERY

1 B – Battery

This lady has undergone a procedure without her consent and to which, had the procedure been abandoned, she would probably not have consented. Battery in principle is a violation of the civil law to touch another person without their consent. The harm resulting from battery does not necessarily have to be physical in nature. In the situation of informed consent harm may be construed as the moral violation of the patient's right to exercise a rational choice.

2 G – Negligence

Battery is not the only legal action that surgeons risk for inadequately respecting their patient's right to informed consent. Although the patient had given his general consent to the surgery in question, he had not been properly advised of its potential hazards (in this case inadvertent damage to other structures by trocar insertion/dissection/diathermy). In such situations, the legal claim is that had the patient known the risks in question, they would not have proceeded with the surgery. NB Surgeons are not protected from accusations of negligence by a signed consent form. Note: in this case, the surgeon might also be deemed negligent for choosing a laparoscopic approach to this surgery in the first place.

3 E – Implied consent

In many situations it is neither necessary nor practicable to give informed (especially written) consent. It is deemed in such situations that the patient's willingness to present themselves for investigation or treatment implies their consent (such as in this case).

4 C – Treatment in best interests under common law

In English law, no one is able to give consent for treatment of another adult against his or her will. The only exception to this rule is treatment of the mental disorder itself in patients sectioned under the 1983 Mental Health Act (answer I). This is *not*, however, true for treatment of other physical conditions in patients with mental illness. However, essential, especially life-saving, treatment may be given to such patients in the patients' best interests under Common Law when they are deemed incapable for any reason to give informed consent.

(Resources for this subject may be obtained from www.doh.gov.uk *and the chapter by Len Doyal in the* Clinical Surgery in General RCS Course *manual.)*

3 LOCAL ANAESTHETICS: TYPES AND DOSAGES

1 G – 56 ml

A 0.25% solution contains 2.5 mg/ml bupivacaine (the number of mg/ml can easily be calculated by multiplying the percentage strength by 10). The maximum safe dose of bupivacaine is 2 mg/kg with or without adrenaline added. Therefore a 70-kg patient can have 140 mg of bupivacaine, which equates to 56 ml of a 0.25% solution (140 ÷ 2.5 = 56).

2 F – 28 ml

A 0.5% solution contains 5 mg/ml lidocaine. The maximum safe dose of lidocaine is 3 mg/kg without adrenaline added and 7 mg/kg with adrenaline. Therefore a 20-kg patient can have 140 mg of lidocaine with adrenaline, which equates to 28 ml of a 0.5% solution (140 ÷ 5 = 28).

3 C – 18 ml

Intravenous regional anaesthesia (IVRA) under tourniquet control is a simple method of providing short-term anaesthesia of the distal arm or leg, first described by August Bier in 1808. The drug of choice for IVRA is prilocaine because it is the least toxic local anaesthetic and has the largest therapeutic index. A 2% prilocaine solution contains 20 mg/ml prilocaine. The maximum safe dose of prilocaine is 6 mg/kg. Therefore a 60-kg patient can have 360 mg of prilocaine, which equates to 18 ml of a 2% solution. NB The pressure in the tourniquet must be constantly observed and maintained at ≥ 50 mmHg above the patient's systolic blood pressure.

4 GENERAL ANAESTHETIC AGENTS

1 K – Suxamethonium

Suxamethonium is a depolarising muscle relaxant that mimics the action of acetylcholine. In this case it was chosen for its rapid onset (as would be required for crash induction). The delay in self-ventilation is known as suxamethonium, or scoline, apnoea. In a normal individual the effects of this agent last for only a few minutes until it has been metabolised by plasma cholinesterase. Deficiency of this enzyme leads to prolonged action, causing apnoea.

2 L – Thiopentone sodium

This is the oldest, cheapest and best understood intravenous induction agent. However, it has been superseded by propofol and etomidate, because of its potential side-effects of marked hypotension, anaphylaxis and bronchospasm. It can also leave patients with a bad hangover. Etomidate is less of a myocardial depressant and is used in patients who have cardiovascular instability. Propofol is the most widely used intravenous agent, allowing for a clear-headed and rapid recovery. It should be used with caution in hypovolaemic patients.

3 F – Halothane

Halothane is a volatile, inhalational anaesthetic, which is well tolerated and non-irritant. It can cause respiratory depression and acts as a negative inotrope. Its major disadvantage, as highlighted by this case, is severe hepatotoxicity (1 in 30,000), with 50% mortality. This is caused when its oxidative metabolites induce immune-mediated hepatic necrosis. As with all inhalational anaesthetics (apart from nitrous oxide), it can be responsible for malignant hyperthermia (1 in 150,000), an inherited autosomal dominant condition. This is therapeutically managed using intravenous dantrolene sodium.

4 I – Nitrous oxide

Nitrous oxide is a potent analgesic, but only a weak anaesthetic. It is used to potentiate the action of other inhalational anaesthetics, allowing a reduction in the dose required. Nitrous oxide will diffuse into any air-containing space, and does so more rapidly than nitrogen. It must not be used in patients who have recently been diving or who have been exposed to high atmospheric pressures, or in patients suspected of having a gas-filled space (eg pneumothorax).

5 COAGULATION DISORDERS

1 G – Protein C deficiency

Protein C stimulates fibrinolysis by destroying activated factors in the coagulation pathway. Its deficiency leads to unchecked coagulation and is the commonest form of hereditary thrombophilia. It is inherited in an autosomal dominant pattern with a variable penetrance. Patients can develop skin necrosis when treated with warfarin because it triggers protein C levels to drop further before the therapeutic inhibition of vitamin K-dependent clotting factors occurs.

2 K – Vitamin K deficiency

A post-operative vitamin K deficiency is not an uncommon haemostatic defect, especially in this particular scenario. Vitamin K is a fat-soluble vitamin absorbed in the terminal ileum with bile salts. Prolonged diarrhoea/high ileostomy output may result in abnormalities of vitamin K absorption. This, combined with treatment with broad-spectrum antibiotics, results in suppression of the normal gut bacterial flora that are in turn an important producer of vitamin K. This condition is best managed with slow intravenous infusion of vitamin K and treatment of the underlying cause of deficiency.

3 D – Haemophilia A

Haemophilia is the commonest hereditary disorder of blood coagulation. The inheritance is sex-linked but 33% of patients have no family history, and presumably result from spontaneous mutations. Haemophilia A is an absence, or low level, of plasma factor VIII, while Haemophilia B (Christmas disease) is the result of a deficiency in factor IX. Clinically the conditions are identical and can only be distinguished on coagulation factor assays. The above presentation is common while recurrent painful haemarthroses and muscle haematomas dominate the clinical picture of severely affected individuals, resulting in progressive deformity. Bleeding episodes are treated with factor VIII replacement or desmopressin. For major surgery, levels are raised to 100% and maintained at 60% until bleeding has ceased.

6 TYPES OF ANAEMIA

1 N – Vitamin B_{12} deficiency

This patient's blood test reveals a macrocytic anaemia. This could have megaloblastic (vitamin B_{12} or folate deficiency) or non-megaloblastic (alcohol, liver disease) causes. Complete resection of the terminal ileum results in the malabsorption of vitamin B_{12} in association with intrinsic factor and bile salts, consequently leading to megaloblastic anaemia, steatorrhoea and diarrhoea. The Schilling test distinguishes between malabsorption of vitamin B_{12} and lack of intrinsic factor. (A megaloblast is a cell in which cytoplasmic and nuclear maturation are out of phase because nuclear maturation is slow.)

2 B – Autoimmune haemolytic anaemia

The blood test reveals a normocytic anaemia of which one of the causes is haemolysis. Haemolysis may result in unconjugated hyperbilirubinaemia, hence jaundice and gallstones, and splenic hypertrophy. Causes are either hereditary or acquired. Acquired haemolysis may be either immune (eg autoimmune – cold or warm antibody-mediated) or non-immune (eg microangiopathic). The direct Coombs' test identifies cells coated with antibody or complement, a positive result indicating an immune cause of haemolysis. Warm autoimmune haemolytic anaemia is associated with other autoimmune disorders, especially systemic lupus erythematosis.

3 H – Iron deficiency

The blood test reveals a microcytic anaemia. One of the commonest causes of which is iron deficiency anaemia, secondary to chronic blood loss. This patient's history should immediately alert you to the possibility of right-sided colonic carcinoma, which frequently results in faecal occult blood loss.

7 BLOOD TRANSFUSION COMPLICATIONS

1 O – Post-transfusion purpura (PTP)

PTP is defined as thrombocytopenia arising 5–12 days after transfusion of red cells. It is associated with the presence in the recipient of antibodies directed against the human platelet antigen (HPA) system. The patient becomes sensitised to foreign platelet antigen (commonly anti-Pl^{A1}), usually as a result of previous pregnancy or, more rarely, transfusion. If the patient then receives subsequent blood carrying this antigen, a secondary response occurs, leading to destruction of the recipient's own platelets. Clinical signs are purpura and mucosal bleeding. Optimal treatment is by means of large doses of intravenous immunoglobulin, or plasma exchange.

2 P – Transfusion-related acute lung injury (TRALI)

This man is suffering from TRALI. This is defined as acute dyspnoea with hypoxia and bilateral pulmonary infiltrates occurring within 24 h of transfusion. When there is no other apparent cause (too delayed to be air embolus) such symptoms point to this as the most likely diagnosis. TRALI is caused by agglutination of the patient's white blood cells when they are exposed to potent HLA antibodies in the blood donor's plasma. Diagnosis is supported by a positive cytotoxic cross-match where the donor's plasma reacts to the patient's white cells. Management consists of supportive measures, such as stopping the transfusion (if the reaction occurs while this is ongoing), resuscitation, oxygen therapy and Intensive Care Unit intervention, with or without ventilation as necessary.

3 K – Immediate haemolytic transfusion reaction

Clinical symptoms of a major transfusion reaction include urticaria, abdominal/lumbar/chest pain, flushing, headache, dyspnoea, vomiting and rigors. Clearly these signs are far easier to elicit in the conscious patient. In this scenario, however, the woman is not able to describe such symptoms. The signs in such a patient are therefore of utmost importance in diagnosing a haemolytic reaction. In the unconscious patient, hypotension (a fall > 10 mmHg) and generalised uncontrollable bleeding are the most important signs. Alongside these, further indications of an immediate haemolytic reaction are fever (an increase of more than 1.5 °C above baseline), jaundice and haemoglobinuria. Immediate haemolytic transfusion reaction is usually the result of ABO incompatibility, leading to complement activation and massive intravascular haemolysis. Most severe reactions occur because of clerical error, hence all documentation should be re-checked and both patient and donor blood (from the bag in use) should undergo repeat cross-matching. The prime objective in the acute management of such a reaction is to maintain blood pressure and renal perfusion. This is achieved by immediate cessation of the transfusion and supportive resuscitation with intravenous fluids, titration of (1 : 10, 000 adrenaline as well as chlorpheniramine (10 mg) and hydrocortisone (100 mg). Renal failure and disseminated intravascular coagulation may lead to death in the worst case scenario.

4 M – Iron overload

Repeated red cell transfusions (often given frequently as prophylaxis to sickle-cell sufferers having regular crises, to suppress haemoglobin S production) can lead to iron overload in the absence of chelation. Each unit of blood contains between 200 and 250 mg of iron. After 12 g of iron have been transfused (approximately 50 units of blood), clinical abnormalities start to appear. Unfortunately, organ damage will have occurred earlier than this. Iron damages the liver, the endocrine organs (leading to failure of growth, delayed or absent puberty, diabetes mellitus, hypothyroidism and hypoparathyroidism) and the myocardium. Parenteral treatment with desferrioxamine can prevent iron overload, if compliance with medication is good. In the absence of intensive iron chelation, death often occurs in the second or third decade, usually from congestive heart failure or cardiac arrhythmias.

Post-operative management and critical care

8 ARTERIAL BLOOD GASES

1 E – Metabolic acidosis and increased anion gap

In an abdominal operation of this duration, the most likely cause of this patient's abnormal arterial blood gases, presenting a few hours post-operatively, is a metabolic acidosis (defined by decreased pH and HCO_3^-) secondary to hypovolaemia. This results in a relative high concentration of serum lactic acid, consequently causing a significant imbalance against serum cations (eg sodium and potassium) producing an increased anion gap. The anion gap is calculated as: $[Na^+] + [K^+] - [Cl^-] - [HCO_3^-]$; so in this patient the anion gap is $138 + 4.0 - 100 - 22 = 20$ mmol/litre (normal range 8–16 mmol/litre). An increased anion gap is the result of an increased concentration of organic acids, as opposed to a metabolic acidosis with a normal anion gap that tends to be the result of a loss of bicarbonate or an ingestion of H^+ ions (eg renal tubular acidosis, pancreatic fistulae).

2 A – Compensated metabolic acidosis

The most likely cause of this patient's symptoms is a missed anastomotic leak, resulting in sepsis, subsequent increased lactic acid production and a consequent metabolic acidosis. The inability of the kidney to excrete the increased acid load shifts the acid–base balance, ie $[H^+] + [HCO_3^-] \leftrightarrow H_2CO_3 \leftrightarrow H_2O + CO_2$, to the right. To compensate for this shift the lungs rapidly respond by increasing the respiratory rate, so reducing CO_2 levels and thereby causing H^+ ions to return toward normal.

3 B – Compensated metabolic alkalosis

A metabolic alkalosis, indicated by raised base excess and serum bicarbonate, can be caused by hydrochloric acid depletion secondary to vomiting. The patient's pH level is at the upper limit of normal and the $p_A(CO_2)$ is raised, indicating respiratory compensation.

4 H – Respiratory acidosis

This patient has developed basal atelectasis and subsequent lower lobe pneumonia, resulting in hypoxia, hypercapnia and resultant respiratory acidosis (pH low, $p_A(O_2)$ low, $p_A(CO_2)$ raised).

9 POST-OPERATIVE HYPOXIA

1 B – Basal atelectasis

Post-operative atelectasis is commonly observed in the early post-operative period, especially after prolonged surgery in the supine position; diaphragmatic dysfunction and reduced surfactant are consequences of general anaesthesia and surgical manipulation that can lead to atelectasis. In addition, inadequate analgesia leads to reduced respiratory excursion and coughing. The resultant hypoventilation of the lung bases leads to localised small airway collapse and is usually accompanied by a low-grade pyrexia.

2 D – Cardiogenic pulmonary oedema

This is the result of either increased hydrostatic pressure (eg volume overload – as in this scenario, and left ventricular failure) or decreased oncotic pressure (eg hypoalbuminaemia). Regardless of aetiology, the fluid accumulates around the lung parenchyma, especially in the dependant basal regions of the lower lobes, causing alveolar collapse.

3 G – Pleural effusion

Fluid in the pleural space can be either a transudate (< 30 g/litre), secondary to either increased hydrostatic pressure (eg from volume overload and left ventricular failure) or decreased oncotic pressure (from hypoalbuminaemia, as in this scenario); or an exudate (> 30 g/litre), secondary to capillary hyperpermeability (from malnutrition, carcinoma, Gram-negative sepsis, etc). Fluid fills the basal aspect of the pleural space, inhibiting gross lung expansion.

4 A – Adult respiratory distress syndrome

Adult respiratory distress syndrome, or non-cardiogenic pulmonary oedema, is often an early manifestation of the systemic inflammatory response syndrome and later development of multi-organ dysfunction. It represents progressive combined ventilatory, perfusion and diffusional pathology. Pulmonary capillary leakage results in impaired oxygen diffusion and reduced lung compliance; additionally leakage into the alveoli produces a hyalination and fibrosis responsible for the characteristic radiological appearance of bilateral pulmonary infiltrates.

10 POST-OPERATIVE PYREXIA

1 F – Chest X-ray

The most likely cause of pyrexia early after surgery is basal atelectasis; indeed, this is the commonest cause of morbidity and mortality in patients following major surgery or trauma. It classically occurs in patients who undergo prolonged surgery in the supine position or in those with inadequate post-operative analgesia. The epidural at T7 is sited too low to provide adequate pain relief. This leads to hypoventilation, decreased clearance of pulmonary secretions, small airway collapse and associated low-grade pyrexia.

2 A – Abdominal ultrasound scan

The most likely cause is either a subhepatic biliary collection, secondary to biliary leakage, or infected haematoma. A simple, safe and cheap investigation is abdominal ultrasound, which also has the advantage of allowing therapeutic guided drainage. Initial treatment also includes fluid resuscitation and broad-spectrum antibiotic therapy.

3 I – Duplex ultrasound scan

The most likely cause of these symptoms is deep vein thrombosis involving the popliteal or femoral vessels. Duplex ultrasonography is the investigation of choice – it is widely available, relatively inexpensive and non-invasive with sensitivity and specificity of 97% and 94%, respectively. Venography, although the gold standard for diagnosis, is reserved for suspected calf vein or iliac vein thrombosis or where a lack of concordance exists between clinical findings, D-dimer assay and/or ultrasonography.

4 J – Exploratory laparotomy

The most likely cause of these symptoms is anastomotic leak. The nature of the surgery performed and the clinical findings suggest this diagnosis. Management involves urgent resuscitation and laparotomy. It carries a significant mortality, and surgery should not be delayed by unnecessary investigations, unless the diagnosis is in doubt.

11 POST-OPERATIVE OLIGURIA

1 A – Acute renal failure (ARF)

This man has suffered ARF as a complication of his aortic aneurysm surgery. The origin of his aneurysm in the scenario is at L2 – around the origin of the renal arteries (L1–L2). Inadvertent damage during surgery or occult embolism, after fresh or organised thrombus is dislodged from the aneurysmal sac, can lead to acute renal failure.

2 B – Cardiogenic shock

This gentleman is diabetic and an arteriopath, as indicated by his admission for vascular bypass surgery. His poor urine output, compromised blood pressure (with no clear evidence of overt or covert haemorrhage) and the vague history of 'indigestion'-type pain that has not settled with antacids, suggest a coronary cause for his hypotension and oliguria. This is confirmed by a failure of fluid bolus replacement to sustain a rise in blood pressure. This man needs thorough cardiovascular assessment (including electrocardiogram, chest X-ray, general bloods, cardiac enzymes and probably central venous pressure measurement). If he has sustained a myocardial infarct clearly he will be unable to undergo thrombolysis: such recent vascular surgery contra-indicates this. Instead treatment should be supportive (oxygen, analgesia), and treatment with inotropes should be initiated if his hypotension fails to improve on the Coronary Care Unit.

12 ENTERAL AND PARENTERAL NUTRITION

1 C – Feeding jejunostomy

Most surgeons will choose to form a feeding jejunostomy at surgery. Feeding is instigated until a gastrograffin swallow demonstrates an intact anastomosis and oral nutrition can be re-instated.

2 E – Low-volume, low-electrolyte feed

This patient will require a low-volume, low-electrolyte feed (ie low sodium and low potassium). The picture of chronic renal failure, which is controlled by continuous ambulatory peritoneal dialysis, means that they will be unable to eliminate high-volume feeds adequately and the resulting fluid overload could precipitate peripheral oedema and cardiac failure. The failed kidneys will be unable to excrete electrolytes efficiently and the low Na^+ and K^+ content in these feeds will prevent dangerous plasma increases in these electrolytes.

3 J – Percutaneous endoscopic gastrostomy (PEG) feeding

It is widely accepted that any patient requiring enteral tube feeding for more than a month should have a more permanent form of feeding tube inserted. This is to prevent the inevitable problems that can occur with chronic use of a naso-enteric tube. Such tubes are associated with considerable patient discomfort; sinusitis and epistaxis are common complications, as are tube-related irritations and blockage. Percutaneous gastrostomy placement is predominantly performed by using either the push or the pull technique. With the push technique, the feeding tube is pushed though the abdominal wall over a wire into the gut using fluoroscopic guidance. Usually, loop catheters or balloon catheters are placed. With the pull technique, the feeding tube is advanced through the patient's mouth into the stomach and pulled out through the abdominal wall by using a snare introduced through a fluoroscopically guided direct gastric puncture site.

4 K – Total parenteral nutrition (TPN)

The average length of the adult human small intestine has been calculated at approximately 600 cm from studies performed on cadavers. Any disease, traumatic injury, vascular accident, or other pathology that leaves less than 200 cm of viable small bowel places the patient at risk for developing short-bowel syndrome and with less than 100 cm, problems are inevitable, especially if there is no colonic absorption of water (as in this case). Clearly nutrition is a significant issue and TPN is almost always required, at least for an initial period. It is sometimes possible to eventually wean to some form of enteral nutrition or use this to supplement home parenteral nutrition.

5 H – Nasojejunal feeding

There is now a wealth of published evidence to support early enteral nutrition in pancreatitis, including severe cases. The basic premise is that feeding helps to maintain the epithelial barrier reducing bacterial translocation and subsequent systemic inflammatory response syndrome/multi-organ dysfunction. While some groups have tried nasogastric feeding in this context, there is usually gastroparesis.

13 ANTI-EMETICS

Vomiting is a complex physiological process that initiates repetitive active contraction of the diaphragm and abdominal muscles to generate a pressure gradient that leads to the forceful expulsion of gastric contents. Nausea and vomiting are primarily controlled by the vomiting centre, which receives input from: (i) ***the chemoreceptor trigger zone*** *(located in the area postrema of the medulla, on the lateral walls of the fourth ventricle, outside the blood–brain barrier); (ii)* ***visceral afferents from the gastro-intestinal tract****, which relay information to the brain regarding gastro-intestinal distension and mucosal irritation; (iii)* ***visceral afferents from outside the gastrointestinal tract*** *(bile ducts, peritoneum, heart and a variety of other organs) (stimulation of such afferents helps explain how 'non-gastrointestinal' pathology may result in vomiting); and (iv)* ***afferents from extramedullary centres in the brain*** *may be stimulated by certain central stimuli (eg odours, fear), vestibular disturbances (motion sickness) and cerebral trauma. Specific receptors that may be targeted include dopamine (D_2), serotonin (5-HT_3), histamine (H_1) and muscarinic (M_1) receptors in the area postrema, H_1 and M_1 receptors in the labyrinths, and 5-HT_3 receptors on peripheral afferents. Many of the anti-emetic drugs act at the level of the chemoreceptor trigger zone. The main classes of anti-emetic agents include: anti-histamine and anti-cholinergic agents, dopamine and serotonin antagonists, and phenothiazines.*

1 E – Prochlorperazine

Phenothiazine compounds, such as prochlorperazine, appear to act primarily through a central anti-dopaminergic mechanism in the chemo-receptor trigger zone. They are of considerable value in the prophylaxis and treatment of post-operative nausea and vomiting, as well as that associated with diffuse neoplastic disease and radiation sickness. Severe dystonic reactions, neuroleptic malignant syndrome and blood dyscrasias are recognised complications. By contrast, benzamide agents, such as metoclopramide, act as dopamine antagonists, not only centrally but also peripherally. In addition, they exert a prokinetic effect on the upper gastro-intestinal tract that contributes to their anti-emetic action.

2 D – Ondansetron

Serotonin antagonists have recently been added to the list of clinically effective anti-emetic agents. Specific 5-HT_3 antagonists such as ondansetron and granisetron have been developed, and appear to act peripherally (on peripheral afferents) and centrally (on the area postrema). They are particularly useful in the treatment of post-operative and post-chemotherapy nausea and vomiting, where they have been most effective compared to placebo and other agents in large randomised trials. The only other class of anti-emetic that acts **both** peripherally and centrally is the benzamides, but the benzamides do **not** exert their peripheral effects on **afferent** neurones, and have a prokinetic effect, differentiating them from the serotonin antagonists.

14 SURGICAL ANALGESIA

1 L – Tramadol

In contrast to other opioids, the analgesic action of tramadol is only partially the result of its inhibition of central μ-receptors. This was demonstrated by the discovery of a monoaminergic activity that inhibits noradrenaline (norepinephrine) and serotonin reuptake, making a significant contribution to the analgesic action by blocking nociceptive impulses at the spinal level. Nevertheless, the affinity for μ-receptors of the central nervous system remains low, being 6000 times lower than that of morphine, so it is of value for treating several pain conditions (step II of the World Health Organisation ladder) where treatment with strong opioids is not required. Tramadol has pharmacodynamic and pharmacokinetic properties that are highly unlikely to lead to dependence.

2 C – Celecoxib

Celecoxib is a selective non-steroidal antinflammatory drug (NSAID) that acts by selective cyclo-oxygenase-2 (COX-2) inhibition to prevent prostaglandin synthesis. It is only licensed for patients with rheumatoid or osteoarthritis. Prostaglandins exert a critical role in the inflammatory process, their synthesis is catalysed by the closely related isozymes, COX-1 and COX-2. The principal pharmacological effect of aspirin and related NSAIDs (eg ibuprufen, diclofenac, naproxen) is the result of their ability to inhibit prostaglandin synthesis by blocking the cyclo-oxygenase activity of both COX-1 and COX-2. COX-1 is responsible for the production of 'housekeeping' prostaglandins that are critical to the maintenance of normal renal function, gastric mucosal integrity and vascular haemostasis; whereas COX-2 promotes the inflammatory pathway. It is suggested that the analgesic, anti-pyretic, anti-inflammatory and anti-thrombogenic actions of NSAIDs were caused by COX-2 inhibition and the unwanted side-effects were the result of inhibition of COX-1. Hence, the development of NSAIDs with greater selectivity for COX-2 receptors. The currently approved COX-2 inhibitors, celecoxib and rofecoxib, are highly selective for COX-2 in comparison with traditional NSAIDs (375-fold and 1000-fold, respectively). Short-term data indicate that the risk of serious upper gastro-intestinal events is lower compared with non-selective NSAIDs; however they do not provide protection against ischaemic cardiovascular events. The National Institute for Clinical Excellence has recommended that cyclo-oxygenase-2 selective inhibitors should only be used in preference to non-selective NSAIDs for patients with a history of peptic ulcer perforation or bleeding; they should also be used in preference to standard NSAIDs for other patients at high risk of developing serious gastro-intestinal side-effects (eg those aged over 65 years, those who are taking other medicines which increase the risk of gastro-intestinal effects, those who are debilitated, or those receiving long-term treatment with maximal doses of standard NSAIDs).

Surgical technique

15 SURGICAL INSTRUMENTS

While perhaps the use of eponyms should not be greatly encouraged in modern clinical practice, it is unlikely that the operating theatre will cease (at least in the near future) to be a 'bastion' of such terminology. Some appreciation is therefore required.

1 E – Eisenhammer retractor

An anal retractor commonly used to assist examination of the ano-rectum under anaesthesia. Alternatives are the Park or Simm retractors.

2 B – Babcock forceps

Babcock's tissue-holding forceps are designed to grasp, rather than crush, contained viscera, thereby avoiding damage and/or possible spillage of contents. Dr W. Wayne Babcock, born in 1872, in addition to writing the most noted textbook of his time, was the inventor of many instruments and techniques in surgery. Other commonly used tissue-holding forceps are Allis, Littlewood and Lane, all of which are traumatic.

3 L – Robert clamp

A variety of ratcheted clamps exist to crush and hold tissue prior for instance to ligation. A Robert clamp is a long, robust and partially curved clamp that is very commonly employed for medium to large structures such as vascular pedicles on the bowel. Smaller, slightly-curved clamps include Dunhill and Mosquito. Examples of more curved clamps (right-angle or greater) are Moynihan and Lloyd Davis (large) and Lahey (smaller).

4 C – Debakey forceps

There are various dissecting forceps that largely differ based on their size and whether they have teeth. Debakey forceps can be straight or angulated and are atraumatic. Adson (small), Gillies (medium) and Officer (large) have teeth and should not be used near vessels or to grasp bowel.

16 SUTURE MATERIALS

Suture materials can be classified in three main ways:

1. *Absorbable or non-absorbable*
2. *Monofilament versus braided*
3. *Natural or synthetic.*

They are also categorised by size.

These qualities confer different properties upon the material. Absorbable sutures give less wound support but also less foreign body reaction than non-absorbable. Monofilaments are less traumatic to tissue but are less easy to handle than braided sutures. Synthetic materials cause less tissue reaction than sutures derived from natural fibres and have generally therefore superseded them.

1 I – PDS

PDS is an absorbable, synthetic monofilament of polydioxanone. It has ideal qualities for use in mass tissue closure, particularly of the abdominal wall. This is because it is predictable and has high tensile strength. It is quoted that PDS retains up to 70% strength at 2 weeks and 50% strength at 4 weeks. It is then completely absorbed in 180–210 days by hydrolysis. Although many surgeons may choose to use nylon for mass closure the attendant risks of sinus formation or stitch extrusion, because of nylon's non-absorbable properties, render this less suitable for such closure. For mass abdominal closure remember the 'four to one' rule. The length of suture used should be four times the length of the wound you are closing. Bites should be taken 1–2 cm apart, and 1–2 cm away from the wound edge to give good closure.

2 M – Steel wire

Steel wire is the material of choice in the closure of sternotomy wounds. It has very high tensile strength and is inert. It may be monofilament or braided and can be very difficult to handle as it kinks easily. It can break and cause pain from sharp ends in the longer term.

3 J – Prolene

Prolene (polypropylene) is a non-absorbable, synthetic monofilament material that is the ideal suture for vascular anastomoses. It is inert, therefore causing minimal tissue reaction, and exerts minimal tissue friction on passage through the vascular endothelium. Braided non-absorbable sutures can also be used, eg Ethibond. This material has an outer layer of polyester to render it smooth, and hence less traumatic to the arterial wall. Use the finest suture strong enough for the job: as a rough guide, 3/0 for the aorta, 4/0 for the iliac arteries, 5/0 for the femoral arteries, 6/0 for the popliteal artery and 7/0 for the tibial arteries are appropriate strengths.

4 J – Prolene

Again, because of its inert and non-absorbable properties, prolene is an excellent choice when siting the polypropylene mesh used in inguinal hernia repairs. Its persistence allows for good positional maintenance of the mesh as patients begin to mobilise in the post-operative period.

17 SURGICAL INCISIONS

1 M – Transverse 'unilateral' Pfannenstiel

This patient has a strangulated femoral hernia that requires urgent surgical repair. The McEvedy (high) approach was classically based on a vertical incision made over the femoral canal and continued upwards above the inguinal ligment; however this frequently resulted in an unsightly scar. This has now been replaced with a transverse 'unilateral' Pfannenstiel incision, which can be extended to form a complete Pfannenstiel incision if a formal laparotomy is required. Alternative approaches include the Lockwood (low), Lothiessen (transinguinal) and laparoscopic approaches. NB Hans Hermann Johannes Pfannenstiel, German gynaecologist (1862–1909).

2 B – Gridiron

The most likely diagnosis in this patient is appendicitis. Appendicectomy is an emergency procedure and the safest incision is a skin-crease modification of the oblique gridiron centred over McBurney's point. It is the Editor's view that attempts at removing the appendix via a Lanz incision can lead to significant peri-operative swelling, especially with a high-lying caecum in an adult, and place the patient at risk. If it is the desperate concern of the surgeon to avoid a visible scar then consideration should be given to performing the case laparoscopically.

3 N – Upper midline

The most likely diagnosis in this patient is a perforated peptic ulcer. In those patients suitable for surgery, access is most commonly by upper midline incision. The historical alternative of a right paramedian incision is now rarely used, providing little additional exposure and potentially rendering part of the abdominal wall anaesthetic and ischaemic with poor wound healing and increased risk of hernias.

18 ON-TABLE POSITIONS

1 E – Lloyd Davies

The patient lies supine on the table, with legs in supports that flex the hips and knees to 45°. The legs can then be separated to allow surgical access to both abdomen and perineum at the same time (as is required during an abdomino-perineal excision of the rectum). To access the pelvis the patient is often also tilted head down, ie Trendelenberg. The lithotomy position is a more exaggerated version of the Lloyd Davies, where hips and knees are flexed to 90°. The lithotomy position was named after the operation that it was historically invented for; the removal of bladder stones. 'Cutting for stone' or lithotomy (*lithos* = stone) was frequently performed by travelling surgeons before the advent of anaesthesia and antisepsis (or fellowships).

2 J – Trendelenberg

In the Trendelenberg position the patient is placed supine, with head-down tilt. This is the most appropriate patient placement for varicose vein surgery as it helps to alleviate pressure in the lower limb venous system and hence decreases intra-operative blood loss. This position can be also be used during laparoscopic pelvic surgery (eg gynaecological intervention, inguinal hernia repair, rectopexy) to keep bowel loops out of the operating field. The reverse Trendelenberg, as it is logically described, adopts a head-up tilt. It is good for use in laparoscopic cholecystectomy/Nissen's fundoplication, where the abdominal contents need to fall away from the region of intervention.

3 C – Lateral decubitus

In the lateral decubitus position the patient is positioned on the contralateral side to their pathology, and the table is flexed in the centre. This stretches the flank of the patient that is uppermost, ie the side of the renal tumour. In this way there is better exposure of the loin between the bony prominences of the ribs and the iliac crest, clearly improving access and operating manoeuvrability.

4 A – Armchair

The seated armchair position is ideal for access to the shoulder, particularly in arthroscopic cases where dependency of the upper limb opens the sub-acromial space. This allows for easier insertion of scope and instruments. In difficult cases it also permits a longitudinal or transverse incision through the deltoid to more fully open up the shoulder joint.

19 LAPAROSCOPIC COMPLICATIONS

1 I – Reduced venous return

Insufflation of the abdomen to create a pneumoperitoneum is important to allow adequate visibility and instrumental access for the surgeon. However, it is not without potential complications. The pressure exerted by the pneumoperitoneum can lead to a reduction in cardiac venous return, resulting in hypotension and a reflex tachycardia. It can also compromise diaphragmatic movement, which is important in patients with restrictive lung disease.

2 A – Abdominal wall emphysema

This is a description of air in the subcutaneous tissues, which can be caused by dissection (pneumodissection) of the fascial planes by carbon dioxide during the formation of a pneumoperitoneum. The dissection of gas into the mediastinum, neck and subcutaneous tissues is very common after laparoscopic anti-reflux surgery. It is managed conservatively, and on clinical and radiological examination a pneumodissection typically resolves within 3 to 4 days.

3 K – Visceral injury: obstruction

The patient has obstructive jaundice. This can occur either as a result of inadvertently clipping the common hepatic or common bile duct (rather than the cystic duct) or because of the presence of a retained stone. Patients with an obstructing gallstone tend to present in the later post-operative course, following resolution of the discomfort associated with surgery.

Management and legal issues

20 BASIC STATISTICS (TAXONOMY)

1 B – χ^2 test

This is the correct test for categorical data, such as male/female, where we wish to establish whether there is a significant difference in proportions between two or more groups (the Fisher's exact test is similar but utilised for only 2 × 2-cell tables with small numbers in each cell). In contrast, *t*-tests, such as the Student's *t*-test (parametric data) and the Mann–Whitney *U*-test (non-parametric data) are used for comparing continuous numerical data.

2 G – The negative predictive value

The proportion of patients with negative test results who are correctly diagnosed is the negative predictive value. In contrast, the proportion of patients with positive test results who are correctly diagnosed is the positive predictive value. Unlike specificity and sensitivity, the positive and negative predictive values give a direct assessment of the usefulness of a test in practice. However in addition, unlike sensitivity and specificity, the positive and negative predictive values are strongly affected by prevalence (ie the proportion of patients with the abnormality). The positive predictive value increases with increasing prevalence and the negative predictive value decreases.

3 F – Likelihood ratio

For any test result, one can compare the probability of getting that result if the patient truly had the disease with the corresponding probability if they were healthy. The ratio of these probabilities is the likelihood ratio, which can be considered to indicate the value of a test for increasing certainty about a positive diagnosis. It is numerically equal to the sensitivity / (1 – specificity).

(Basic resources for this subject may be obtained from the chapter by Hugh Dudley in the Clinical Surgery *in General RCS Course manual or, for the more avid student, from a book entitled* Practical Statistics for Medical Research *by Douglas G Altman.)*

21 TYPES OF SCIENTIFIC EVIDENCE

1 H – Meta-analysis

When reviewing the impact of new therapies, evidence can come from several studies of modest size and with slightly differing conclusions. One solution might be to carry out a definitive randomised controlled trial but this might require considerable time, effort and expense. An alternative is to combine data from several modest studies into a meta-analysis. By combining studies in a coherent (statistically robust) way, conclusions can be reached on a larger pool of subjects.

2 C – Cohort study

This differs slightly from a randomised controlled trial in that it generally takes two or more large cohorts of subjects (rather than a specific sample size of patients) and follows them up long term for the effects of a certain agent, eg an environmental factor on the basis of which they are selected. An example is Sir Richard Doll's work associating lung cancer with smoking by observing a cohort of 40,000 doctors in four cohorts according to number of cigarettes smoked over 10 years.

3 B – Case series

This is synonymous with a series of case reports which together illustrate an interesting aspect of a condition or treatment. Although they are not randomised, are rarely prospective, and represent a low relative weight in the traditional hierarchy of evidence, they are easy for the less scientifically minded to digest and can still convey very important information rapidly before a definitive trial can be performed, eg McBride's 1961 case series of two infants with limb absence born to mothers taking Thalidomide first alerted the world to this terrible drug complication.

(Resources for this subject may be obtained from the BMJ book by Trisha Greenhalgh entitled How to read a paper.*)*

22 PRINCIPLES OF TRIAL DESIGN AND CONDUCT

1 R – Type II error

This is the definition of a term used in the context of hypothesis testing. A type I error in contrast is one in which we reject the null hypothesis when a real difference is not present. These terms are most commonly cited in the context of study design where the probability of type I and II errors can be reduced by performing a prior power analysis in which the correct sample size is estimated on the basis of setting α and β values which represent the probabilities that a type II and type I error will be committed. NB the null hypothesis is the cornerstone of hypotheticodeductive reasoning (Karl Popper) not a term describing a negative approach to research!

2 D – Exclusion bias

This is one of the four components of systematic bias (the others are in the list) that should be eliminated/minimised by good trial design and conduct. So-called 'drop outs' or exclusions from trials can occur for many reasons and can introduce bias quite easily since the tendency (even unintentially) is to exclude participants to favour the outcome of the trial. Where exclusions occur, this problem can be reduced by analysis on an 'intention to treat' basis (ie they are still included in the analysis).

3 G – Minimisation

This is an alternative to simple randomisation (the commonest method used to reduce selection bias) when this might potentially introduce large differences in the characteristics of comparison groups within a trial. Other methods include stratified randomisation but this is usually used for single binary variables such as sex.

(Resources for this subject may be obtained from the BMJ book by Trisha Greenhalgh entitled How to read a paper.*)*

23 SCIENTIFIC RESEARCH TECHNIQUES

1 C – DNA microarray

DNA microarray, or DNA chips, are fabricated by high-speed robotics, generally on glass but sometimes on nylon substrates, for which probes with known identity are used to determine complementary binding, so allowing massively parallel gene expression and gene discovery studies. An experiment with a single DNA chip can provide researchers with information on thousands of genes simultaneously.

2 L – Western blotting

Blotting is a descriptive term for the transfer of molecules out of a gel and onto a filter membrane by a wicking action, although the term is now used for electrotransfers or vacuum transfers. In the original description of blotting, Dr Edwin Southern developed the technique to make the gel-resolved nucleic acid more accessible to subsequent manipulation, such as identification by hybridisation – this was Southern blotting. Northern and Western blotting followed the original nomenclature (perhaps not very helpfully). In Western blotting proteins are separated on a gel, and blotted (by electrophoretic transfer) then detected with antibodies specific to the protein of interest. Northern blotting is the similar separation and blotting of RNA antibodies to RNA.

3 H – The polymerase chain reaction (PCR)

This is a relatively well-established technique that has revolutionised many aspects of molecular biology. It amplifies DNA to produce adequate amounts for subsequent use. Two synthetic oligonucleotide primers, typically 20–25 nucleotides in length and complementary to the flanking region of the target sequence to be amplified, are orientated 5′ to 3′. They are hybridised to opposite strands of the target sequence and extended using thermally stable DNA polymerases until the region between the two primers is completely replicated. Initial hybridisation of the two oligonucleotides requires heat denaturation of the double-stranded DNA template. The temperature is then lowered to an optimum at which primers anneal to their complementary sequences. Finally, polymerase elongation, again requiring an optimal temperature, completes the synthesis which effectively results in doubling the concentration of the target DNA segment. This cycle is repeated for 25–35 rounds using commercially available thermal cyclers.

4 A – Cloning

This technology has been widely used since the 1970s, and has become a common practice in molecular biology laboratories today. To clone a gene, a DNA fragment containing the gene of interest is isolated from chromosomal DNA using restriction enzymes and then united with a plasmid that has been cut with the same restriction enzymes. When the fragment of chromosomal DNA is joined with its cloning vector in the laboratory it is called a recombinant DNA molecule. Following introduction into suitable host cells, the recombinant DNA can then be reproduced along with the host cell DNA to produce sufficient quantity for further studies.

(Resources for this subject may be obtained from the book by Bradley, Johnson & Rubenstein entitled Lecture notes on molecular medicine.*)*

24 THE LANGUAGE OF THE NEW NHS

The Editor apologises for the inclusion of this question. However, it is a sad fact that all of us involved in the delivery of health care (even including surgeons) within the New NHS require some understanding of the current language of health-care delivery. Such questions are also a favourite of SpR interview panels!

1 G – National service frameworks (NSFs)

These, in addition to setting national standards, also put in place strategies to support implementation and ensure progress within a reasonable timescale. It is aimed that there will be one new framework per year and they include goals for common and important diseases such as coronary heart disease and cancer. They differ from 'National Targets', which address politically 'hotter potatoes' such as waiting times.

2 L – Primary-care trusts (PCTs)

These new organisations described in the NHS plan (2000) are gradually replacing the existing primary-care groups (PCGs) which were previously established under The New NHS (1997) and Health Act (1999) and whose role was similar but only included health-care workers. These themselves are now being usurped by 'Care Trusts' in New NHS parlance. PCTs are advised but not controlled by the Strategic Health Authorities (SHAs).

3 B – Clinical governance

Beloved of interviews and vivas, this definition is as verbose as it is unhelpful. In reality, clinical governance encompasses a range of clinical activities aimed at improving safety for patients. Originally, it had three components: clinical audit, adverse incident reporting and continued professional development. It is now said (presumably in a link to wisdom) to have seven 'pillars' (even Islam has only five) that are clinical audit, clinical risk management, learning effectiveness, patient experience effectiveness, communication effectiveness, resource effectiveness and strategic effectiveness.

Clinical microbiology

25 SURGICALLY IMPORTANT MICRO-ORGANISMS

1 P – *Staphylococcus aureus*

The likely organism is *Staphylococcus aureus,* which is the most common cause of wound infection. It is a Gram-positive coccus that classically causes suppuration, particularly skin abscesses. It may cause cellulitis that is clinically indistinguishable from that caused by *Streptococcus pyogenes.* Coliforms rarely cause wound infection except in synergy with anaerobes such as *Bacteroides* and are more common following colorectal surgery.

2 M – *Pasteurella multocida*

Pasteurella multocida is a Gram-negative parvobacterium. It is a common pathogen, found in the majority of animal bites. Other less common organisms include *Staphylococcus aureus, Streptococcus pyogenes, Eikenella corrodens* and other anaerobes that are commensal in animal mouths. Human mouths contain an even wider range of organisms. Treatment will therefore need to cover all of these pathogens and could typically include augmentin or an oral cephalosporin with metronidazole on an empirical basis until results of the swab are known.

3 F – *Escherichia coli*

This is a Gram-negative, facultative (ie can grow without oxygen) anaerobic bacillus and is the most likely cause of this gentleman's infection. The other possible pathogens include *Proteus, Pseudomonas aeruginosa, Klebsiella, Enterococcus* and *Staphylococcus aureus.* Fewer than 10^3 organisms/ml of urine are not considered significant. More than 10^5 organisms/ml in pure culture are diagnostic.

26 COMPLICATIONS OF TUBERCULOSIS

*Tuberculosis (TB) is caused by an aerobic bacillus (*Mycobacterium tuberculosis*), which has a waxy coat that appears red with acid-fast stains. It is distinctive from other granulomatous diseases, such as sarcoidosis, by its necrotising (caseating) granulomatous tissue response. Transmission, via inhalation of infected droplets, results in Primary Pulmonary Tuberculosis or a Ghon complex. This consists of a Ghon focus in the lung periphery with an associated draining lymph node that may be asymptomatic. Reactivated, or Secondary, Pulmonary Tuberculosis, results in an active infection typically in the apex of the lung, known as an Assman lesion. Either stage can progress to form tuberculous bronchopneumonia or spread more distally to a number of organs, causing miliary tuberculosis.*

1 F – Meningitis

In human immunodeficiency virus infection, patients frequently have florid infections with both *Mycobacterium tuberculosis* and other forms of mycobacterium (*M. avium* and *M. intracellulare*), which are opportunistic pathogens. Other neurological manifestations of miliary TB include diffuse encephalitis, brain abscesses (tuberculomas) or cranial or peripheral neuropathy.

2 G – Osteomyelitis

This gentleman has signs of acute spinal cord compression, which within the context of this question, is secondary to the presence of a tuberculous abscess in his spine. This constitutes a surgical emergency. The bone is weakened by the presence of pus that spreads inwards into the extra-dural space and outwards into the paraspinal tissue. Often the patient is left with a kyphosis, known as Pott's disease. Sir Percival Pott (1714–1788) was an English surgeon of St Bartholomew's Hospital, London. Pott lent his name to a variety of pathologies, not least a type of ankle fracture involving the distal fibula, which he described after sustaining the said injury himself after falling off a horse.

3 K – Scrofula (cervico-facial TB)

Scrofula is common in undiagnosed, neglected cases of TB, and patients present with multiple, tender, matted, posterior or supra-clavicular lymph nodes that lie deep to the deep fascia. These may begin to point through the deep fascia into the subcutaneous plane resulting in a 'collar-stud' abscess, so named because of the two adjacent abscesses that communicate via a narrow tract. The overlying skin temperature is normal because the caseating process is slow, so there is little or no hyperaemia, resulting in a 'cold abscess'.

27 APPROPRIATE ANTI-MICROBIAL THERAPY

1 H – Imipenem

This ventilated patient is a good candidate for opportunistic infections, and in this case the pathogen is *Pseudomonas aeruginosa,* a Gram-negative bacillus. It is also a common and often deadly pathogen in patients with cystic fibrosis and in burns victims. In this patient colonisation of the airway and endo-tracheal tube results in low-grade bronchopneumonia. Antibiotic therapy needs to account for the previous administration of a penicillin, cephalosporin and metronidazole. Therefore the use of a broader-spectrum agent such as imipenem, ciprofloxacin, or tazocin would be appropriate.

2 N – Vancomycin

The use of cephalosporins promotes the proliferation of gut *Clostridium difficile,* which causes pseudomembranous colitis. The exotoxin produced results in damage to the gut epithelial cell membrane with resultant ulceration and breach of the mucosal barrier. This can cause pyrexia, blood loss and loose, distinctive smelling diarrhoea. Identification of the *C. difficile* toxin can be performed rapidly, in most laboratories, using a latex screening test. Treatment involves stopping the causative antibiotic and fluid resuscitation. The patient should also be barrier nursed until the diarrhoea has settled for at least 48 hours. Appropriate antibiotic therapy includes oral metronidazole or vancomycin.

3 F – Flucloxacillin

The most likely organism causing this septic arthritis is *Staphylococcus aureus,* and as described, this lady would require urgent drainage and wash-out of her knee joint. A full septic screen is always required prior to commencement of any empirical treatment in such cases, since anti-microbial resistance and subsequent sterile cultures can complicate therapy. Flucloxacillin treatment would be appropriate here provided resistance is not present.

28 STERILISATION AND DISINFECTION

1 G – Ethylene oxide

Sterilisation is described as the complete destruction of all viable micro-organisms. Heat-sensitive equipment, sutures and other single-use items are prepared using ethylene dioxide as part of an industrial process. The gas is toxic but effective at killing vegetative spores, bacteria and viruses.

2 I – Glutaraldehyde

Joseph Lister pioneered the concept of antisepsis in 1867 while he was Professor of Surgery at the Glasgow Royal Infirmary. He was able to reduce post-operative infections with the use of carbolic acid spray. Modern day antiseptic techniques have now moved on but the essential principles are the same. Disinfection is defined as a reduction in the number of viable organisms and is synonymous with antisepsis except that disinfectants are used in non-living tissue. Glutaraldehyde is rapidly active against bacteria and viruses including hepatitis B virus and human immunodeficiency virus but is less effective against spores and *Mycobacterium tuberculosis*. However, steam with formaldehyde (another more toxic aldehyde) can be used as a method of sterilisation.

3 B – Autoclave

Autoclaving is a sterilisation technique that uses saturated steam at high pressure and kills all organisms including heat-resistant spores, *Mycobacterium tuberculosis* and viruses. The holding time describes the minimum amount of time at a set temperature that guarantees sterility. The Bowie–Dick test is the colour change seen on a strip of heat-sensitive tape (diagonally-striped) attached to wrapped instruments that monitors steam penetration associated with the sterilisation process. Each use of the autoclave is documented in a printout that is, however, the only absolute method of guaranteeing sterility.

Emergency medicine/trauma

29 TYPES OF SHOCK

1 B – Cardiogenic

This patient has Beck's classic triad of tachycardia, muffled heart sounds and engorged neck veins with hypotension resistant to fluid therapy suggesting cardiac tamponade. Cardiac tamponade, a well-recognised cause of cardiogenic shock, results in impairment of cardiac function and effective failure of the heart to maintain the circulation by 'pump failure'. It has a 90% mortality, prompt pericardiocentesis providing the only relief.

2 E – Class 3 haemorrhagic

This patient most likely has a leaking abdominal aortic aneurysm associated with a 30–40% blood volume loss (approximately 2000 ml in a 70-kg adult). Patients with this volume of blood loss almost always present with the classic signs of inadequate peripheral perfusion, marked tachycardia and tachypnoea, significant changes in mental status, and a measurable fall in systolic pressure. Management includes urgent fluid resuscitation, blood transfusion and emergency surgical repair.

3 K – Septic

This patient has developed septic shock. Circulating endotoxins, commonly from Gram-negative organisms, produce vasodilatation – producing a widened pulse pressure and warm peripheries – and impair energy utilisation at a cellular level. Tissue hypoxia can occur even with normal or high oxygen delivery rates because of increased tissue oxygen demands and direct impairment of cellular oxygen uptake. In addition, the endotoxin causes capillary wall hyperpermeability, worsened by the stimulation of proteolytic enzymes, leading to poorly controlled fluid transfer from the intravascular to the interstitial space, effectively resulting in hypovolaemia. The situation is aggravated by the negatively inotropic effect of bacterial endotoxin on the myocardium.

30 DRUGS USED IN CRITICAL CARE

1 G – Dobutamine

Dobutamine stimulates both β_1- and β_2-receptors. Stimulation of β_1-receptors produces a good cardiac inotropic and chronotropic response, leading to improved cardiac output, and stimulation of β_2-receptors produces a degree of vasodilatation, especially in skeletal muscle ('inodilatation'). Dobutamine can be used in combination with noradrenaline if sepsis and hypotension are a problem. Studies have demonstrated that dobutamine is more effective than dopamine (dosage-dependent roles, for example at low doses it is a D_{1A}-agonist, at intermediate doses β_1-adrenoreceptor effects appear, and at high doses α_1-effects predominate) when improvements in oxygen delivery [$D(O_2)$] and uptake [$V(O_2)$] are considered.

2 D – Amrinone

Amrinone (and enoximone) are phosphodiesterase III inhibitors that increase intracellular cyclic AMP. They improve hypotension, principally caused by cardiogenic shock, by their dual action of increasing cardiac output and decreasing systemic vascular resistance ('inodilatation'). The addition of dobutamine is considered to be synergistic.

3 L – Noradrenaline

Noradrenaline stimulates α_1-adrenoreceptors with minor β_1- and β_2-effects. It is employed conventionally when increased systemic vascular resistance (to increase the blood pressure by increasing left ventricular after-load) is required to maintain the mean arterial pressure after fluid replacement and dobutamine infusion have proved inadequate. This is commonly the case in septic shock where inflammatory mediator activation causes systemic vasodilatation.

31 PRIORITIES IN IMMEDIATE TRAUMA CARE

1 A – Airway management

Regardless of the presentation of the patient, the management of this man follows the Advanced Trauma Life Support (ATLS) criteria of Airways, Breathing and Circulation. It appears that he has sustained oro-facial trauma, and possibly aspirated. He needs oropharyngeal suction and insertion of an appropriate airway. Once his breathing has been managed, intravenous access must be gained to begin fluid resuscitation. He demonstrates signs of Class II haemorrhagic shock (15–30% blood loss).

2 I – Pericardiocentesis

This lady has signs of cardiac tamponade, although a differential diagnosis would have included tension pneumothorax had she demonstrated unequal air entry. Cardiac tamponade results in the classic Beck's triad of raised jugular venous pressure, muffled heart sounds and hypotension. There would also be a resultant pulsus paradoxus or a large fall in systolic pressure and blood volume on inspiration. Her hypotension is secondary to a low cardiac output because of ineffectual myocardial contraction. Immediate pericardiocentesis is necessary, which involves insertion of a broad-bore needle, attached to a three-way syringe, into a point 1–2 cm inferior to the left of the xiphochondral junction. The needle should be advanced slowly, while aspirating, towards the tip of the left scapula, while carefully observing the electrocardiogram trace for evidence of a 'current of injury', eg extreme ST-T waves or widened QRS complexes. This alerts the operator to the fact that the needle has been inserted into the myocardium.

3 G – Intravenous access and fluid resuscitation

This man has clear signs of Class IV haemorrhagic shock. This is seen following blood loss of more than 2 litres (> 40%) and results in drowsiness and, occasionally, aggression. Class IV haemorrhagic shock is classified as a pulse rate > 140/min, decreased blood pressure and pulse pressure, and a respiratory rate > 35 breaths/min. The likely source of bleeding is from within the abdomen and a possible long-bone fracture of his lower limb, both of which will also require attention. However, he requires management according to the A,B,C principles of ATLS, with specific management of his circulation. In the initial stages, in casualty, this involves crystalloid fluid replacement followed promptly by blood therapy.

32 MANAGEMENT DECISIONS IN TRAUMA CARE

1 D – Computed tomography (CT) scan

The CT scanner is also known as the 'doughnut of death' to many trauma surgeons, highlighting the need for a stable patient, an appropriate accompanying team and adequate resuscitation facilities in the imaging unit. Often this is not the case, making management decisions difficult. If in doubt about your facilities, then it would be prudent to consider other options, including proceeding to theatre. If the patient demonstrates any signs of compromise prior to transfer then delay doing so until resuscitation has been completed. This gentleman appears to have signs of intra-abdominal trauma but is currently stable. Despite its drawbacks, CT imaging is excellent for assessing the extent of organ damage, retroperitoneal injury and pelvic organ injury and in therefore assisting decision-making regarding operative intervention. It has an accuracy of 92–98% but can miss small diaphragmatic and bowel injuries.

2 F – Emergency laparotomy

Despite the evidence of a significant head injury, this gentleman's immediate threat to life is hypovolaemia from an ongoing intra-abdominal bleed. This is likely to originate from his spleen, and is not improving despite resuscitation. The 'tap' must be turned off and he needs to undergo an emergency laparotomy. A FAST scan would confirm free fluid (and would routinely be performed in units with a radiologist in the trauma team); however, it would not influence management. The patient should not have a CT scan until after laparotomy.

Increased availability of imaging techniques (CT and FAST scans) has led to a decline in the use of diagnostic peritoneal lavage. However, its application continues to be described in the ATLS guidelines for both haemodynamically stable and unstable patients. The Editor's view is that it has a role in the haemodynamically unstable with a negative FAST scan where doubt exists regarding laparotomy but where a CT scan is contra-indicated.

3 G – Emergency thoracotomy

This man was suffering from a massive haemothorax (with a bit of pneumothorax). The chest drain resolves the respiratory embarrassment but fails to help the haemorrhage, which is on-going. Thoracotomy is indicated if a surgeon, qualified by training and experience, is present in the following scenarios:

- > 1500 ml blood drains immediately
- > 200 ml/h blood drains for > 2–4 h
- persistent transfusions
- penetrating anterior trauma medial to the nipple, or posteriorly, medial to the scapula.

It should be performed in theatre with full equipment. NB This procedure differs from a resuscitation thoracotomy (ie one performed in The Emergency Department), which has only two indications:

- penetrating chest injury with witnessed cardiac arrest of < 5 min duration
- uncontrolled life-threatening haemorrhage with tracheo-bronchial bleeding.

33 THE RED EYE

1 K – Scleritis

The sclera and episclera can both become inflamed in autoimmune conditions, particularly rheumatoid arthritis. Unlike conjunctivitis, inflammation of these layers of the eye produces a localised region of injection. The distinction between episcleritis and scleritis is related to severity of symptoms and potential complications. Scleritis is characteristically much more painful than episcleritis, and the signs of inflammation are more extensive. It may ultimately result in ocular perforation. All patients require opthalmological review, and steroid eye drops will provide symptomatic relief and hasten recovery.

2 A – Acute closed-angle glaucoma

This scenario depicts a typical presentation of acute closed-angle glaucoma. This includes the rapid onset of pain, characteristically in the evening, when the pupil becomes semi-dilated (light intensity decreases). Prior episodes that have been relieved by sleep, when the pupil constricts, are also distinctive in this disease. In acute closed-angle glaucoma apposition of the lens to the back of the iris prevents the flow of aqueous from the posterior chamber to the anterior chamber. Accumulation of aqueous behind the iris pushes it forwards on to the trabecular meshwork, preventing normal drainage of aqueous from the eye. This causes an acute rise in intraocular pressure, requiring emergency intervention to preserve sight. Acetazolamide given intravenously and pilocarpine eye drops should be rapidly administered until definitive surgical/laser decompression can be achieved.

3 H – Hyphaema

Blood in the anterior chamber of the eye is known as a hyphaema. Commonly resulting from blunt trauma to the globe, this must be treated as an emergency as further bleeding may increase intraocular pressure and compromise sight. Other important sequelae of blunt ocular trauma are also demonstrated in this case. When the eye itself absorbs impact, transmitted forces to the orbit can result in a 'blow-out' fracture, particularly of the thin orbital floor. Clues to such an occurrence include diplopia, defective eye movements (related to inferior rectus muscle prolapse through the fracture site), emphysema (fracture through a sinus) and recession of the eye (enophthalmus).

4 C – Anterior uveitis

Inflammation of the iris and ciliary body is known as anterior uveitis. At-risk groups for such disorders include those with seronegative arthropathies, particularly if they are positive for HLA-B27 histocompatability antigen (in this case the young man has symptoms of ankylosing spondylitis). Other causes include sarcoidosis, and several infections such as herpes zoster ophthalmicus, syphilis and tuberculosis. It is important to treat the underlying cause and ensure that there is no disease in the rest of the eye that is giving rise to signs of an anterior uveitis (including more posterior inflammation, a retinal detachment, or an intraocular tumour).The pupil is irregular because of adhesions of the iris to the lens (posterior synechiae). Topical steroids help to reduce inflammation.

34 ACUTE LOSS OF VISION

1 D – Giant cell (temporal) arteritis

This scenario demonstrates the classical presentation of someone afflicted with giant cell arteritis. The patient often notices scalp tenderness (often on combing the hair on the affected side), with concurrent visual loss and malaise. They may also report pain on chewing (jaw claudication) and shoulder pain. There is an association with polymyalgia rheumatica. An erythrocyte sedimentation rate (ESR) greater than 40 is highly suggestive of the disease (and there are very few other diagnoses with an ESR > 100). Be aware that a temporal artery biopsy may miss the affected section of artery as the disease can skip regions of vascular endothelium. A strong history should prompt the commencement of oral or intravenous high-dose steroid therapy (even prior to biopsy and its results). Steroids will not restore visual loss but will prevent loss of sight in the other eye.

2 O – Retinal detachment

Retinal detachment can occur in 1 : 10, 000 of the normal population. The probability is increased in people who are short-sighted (myopes); have undergone cataract surgery, as in this specific case, (particularly if this was complicated by vitreous loss); have suffered from a detached retina in the other eye; or who have been subjected to recent severe eye trauma. Symptoms of posterior vitreous detachment, including 'floaters' (pigment or blood in the vitreous) and flashing lights (retinal traction), may precede the onset of retinal detachment itself. As the condition progresses, the patient notices the development of a visual field defect, often likened to a 'shadow' or 'curtain' coming down. If a superior detachment occurs this field defect can evolve rapidly. If the macula becomes detached there is a marked fall in visual acuity.

3 N – Retinal artery occlusion

Retinal artery occlusion is usually embolic in nature. The three main forms of emboli are: fibrin-platelet emboli (from diseased carotids, as in this case); cholesterol emboli (from diseased carotids) and calcific emboli (from diseased heart valves). The presentation can vary but often the patient complains of sudden painless loss of all or part of the vision. In this scenario the fleeting loss of vision experienced by the patient is caused by the fibrin–platelet emboli obstructing, and then passing through, the retinal circulation (amaurosis fugax). Symptoms, therefore, persist for a few minutes then dissipate. Cholesterol and calcific emboli (which are less pliant) may result in permanent obstruction of the retinal vessel, with no visual recovery. On fundoscopic examination the acutely affected retina is oedematous (swollen, pale), while the fovea remains red (cherry red spot) as it has no supply from the retinal circulation. Acute management of the condition is aimed at dilating the arteriole to encourage passage of the embolus. Results are often disappointing (although better if the patient is seen within 24 h of the onset of obstruction). Intravenous acetazolamide (reducing intra-ocular pressure), ocular massage (to exert pressure on vessels in an attempt to dislodge the embolus), anterior chamber paracentesis (to release aqueous and rapidly lower intra-ocular pressure) and carbon dioxide re-breathing (vasodilatory effects) are therapeutic techniques that can be employed. The patient should be thoroughly investigated for systemic vascular disease.

Principles of oncology

35 CHEMOTHERAPEUTIC AGENTS

1 M – Oxaliplatin

Oxaliplatin belongs to a new class of platinum agents. It contains a platinum atom complexed with oxalate and diaminocyclohexane (DACH). The exact mechanism of action of oxaliplatin is not known. Oxaliplatin forms reactive platinum complexes, which are believed to inhibit DNA synthesis by forming inter-strand and intra-strand cross-linking of DNA molecules. Pre-clinical studies have shown oxaliplatin to be synergistic with 5-fluorouracil.

2 D – Cyclophosphamide

Cyclophosphamide, an alkylating agent, is consistently used in all combination chemotherapy regimens. Combination regimens are superior to single agents in the adjuvant setting. The Oxford Overview analysis and other large randomised trials have shown slight, but statistically significant, superiority of anthracycline-containing regimens (eg doxorubicin, an anti-tumour antibiotic, and cyclophosphamide) over traditional CMF (cyclophosphamide, methotrexate and 5-fluorouracil – the latter two are anti-metabolites). Adjuvant chemotherapy results in an approximately 25% decrease of breast cancer mortality. However, the determination of the anthracycline-containing regimen of choice is still under investigation. Cyclophosphamide causes prevention of cell division primarily by cross-linking DNA strands. It is cell-cycle phase non-specific.

3 J – Goserelin acetate

Goserelin acetate is a luteinising hormone-releasing hormone (LHRH) agonist (unlike flutamide which is an androgen antagonist). Non-surgical management of prostate cancer involves a programme of regular clinical (with rectal) examination and prostatic specific antigen monitoring. It is considered in patients of advanced age or those who have significant life-limiting co-morbidities and a life expectancy of less than 15 years. Androgen ablation is used in situations in which patients are unwilling to undergo potentially curative treatment options yet want some form of treatment above watchful waiting. Androgen ablation can be performed in multiple ways, such as using LHRH agonists and antagonists or oral anti-androgens (steroidal and non-steroidal).

4 H – 5-Fluorouracil

This anti-metabolite is usually used in combination with folinic acid (Leucovorin). There is very good evidence now for its use in the adjuvant setting for Dukes C tumours and some evidence for use in high-risk Dukes B tumours. Regimens may also include irinotecan and oxaliplatin. It now exists in an oral form (Capecitabine), which is expensive but obviously advantageous.

36 CAUSES OF PAIN IN PALLIATIVE CARE

1 C – Capsular stretching

Colorectal cancer cells primarily metastasise to the liver via the portal venous system. They quickly develop an arterial blood supply and grow at a variable rate in discrete spherical masses, varying from one to dozens. Many lodge near the surface of the liver, and when their growth reaches the liver capsule they cause stretching and unremitting pain. Pain control is typically step-wise, commencing with paracetamol, then codeine-based analgesics, until morphine or diamorphine is required. Non-steroidal anti-inflammatory drugs often have an excellent additive effect in this situation; steroids can reduce swelling, inflammation and pain, dexamethasone being the drug of choice.

2 N – Spinal cord compression

Advanced prostate cancer results from any combination of lymphatic, blood, or contiguous local spread. Manifestations of metastatic and advanced prostate cancer may include anaemia, bone marrow suppression, weight loss, pathological fractures, spinal cord compression, pain, haematuria, ureteral and/or bladder outlet obstruction, urinary retention, chronic renal failure, urinary incontinence, and symptoms relating to bony or soft-tissue metastases. Elderly patients presenting in the emergency department with sudden onset of weakness of the legs with a history of prostate cancer should raise the suspicion of spinal cord compression. Neurological examination, including determination of external anal sphincter tone, should be performed to help detect spinal cord compression. Treatment involves emergency spinal cord decompression.

3 K – Peripheral nerve compression

The patient's buttock sarcoma is compressing the sciatic nerve, mimicking sciatica secondary to lumbar disc protusion. Generally, soft-tissue tumours grow centripetally, most respect fascial boundaries and hence remain confined to the compartment of origin until later stages of disease. Once the tumour reaches the anatomic limits of the compartment, it is more likely to breach compartmental boundaries. Major neurovascular structures are usually compressed as opposed to being enveloped or invaded by tumour, causing localised symptoms. Pain produced by nerve compression or an infiltrating tumour is termed neuropathic. Treatment involves resection if possible, if not a trial of opioids is worthwhile, usually in conjunction with an adjuvant analgesic. Adjuvant analgesics are drugs with a primary indication other than pain (eg anti-convulsants and anti-depressants) but are analgesic in some painful conditions. Neurolytic blocks may be considered if patients fail to respond to pharmacological agents. Non-drug methods are used in conjunction with drug treatment but not all patients find them helpful. Most rely on counter-irritation and range from systematic rubbing of the affected part, through application of heat, cold, or chemicals, to acupuncture or transcutaneous electrical nerve stimulation.

37 CANCER STAGING

1 A – Breslow staging

The two main staging systems for histologically assessing the invasion of malignant melanoma are Breslow's depth of invasion and Clark's level of invasion. Breslow's stage (A. Breslow, 1970) records the actual measurement (in millimetres) of the depth of lesion, using the micrometer on the microscope. Clark's staging (W.H. Clark *et al.*, 1969) requires excision of the entire lesion and is based on the histological layers of the skin (eg epidermis, papillary dermis, reticular dermis). It has five levels (I–V). NB Neither Breslow's or Clark's staging assesses lymph node involvement or distant metastases.

2 K – T_3, N_2, M_0

The TNM (tumour, nodes, metastases) scoring system is used widely to stage most cancers. It is based on histological assessment of the resected tumour and associated lymph nodes, along with imaging techniques that look for metastatic deposits. The colorectal TNM staging classification was last revised in 1997. The tumour (T) element of the classification looks at depth of invasion of the tumour into and through the colon (T_3 signifies penetration through muscularis propria into subserosa (if present), or peri-colic fat but not into the peritoneal cavity or other organs). The nodes (N) element assesses the number and site of nodes involved (N_2 represents four or more peri-colic/peri-rectal nodes containing disease).The metastasis (M) aspect is generally assessed by imaging techniques, although intra-operative findings such as liver metastases are relevant (M_0 means no distant metastases).

3 C – Dukes A

The original Dukes' system was used to describe rectal carcinomas but can also be applied to carcinomas of the colon. This amazing work (Cuthbert Dukes and St Marks Hospital, 1932) that clearly demonstrated the relationship of stage and grade to prognosis, also alluded to the adenoma–carcinoma sequence and to the need for screening for polyps. Stage A tumours were defined as those limited to the wall (not extending beyond muscularis propria), stage B as those extending through the wall (into subserosa and/or serosa, or extra-rectal tissues), and stage C as those having lymph node involvement. The stage C was later subdivided by Dukes himself into C1, when only peri-rectal nodes are positive, and C2, when nodes at the point of mesenteric blood vessel ligature (called apical nodes) are involved. The TNM system, while more cumbersome, confers more information but the simplicity of Dukes maintains its popularity (both are now usually included in pathology reporting).

4 F – Gleason 6

The Gleason grading system is the most commonly used prostate cancer grading system. It involves assigning numbers (a Gleason grade) to cancerous prostate tissue assessed histologically. The numerical range (from 1 to 5) is based on how much the arrangement of the cancer cells mimics the way normal prostate cells form glands. Two grades are assigned to the two most common patterns of cells that appear; these two grades (which can be the same or different) are then added together to determine the Gleason score (ranging from 1 to 10). An overall score of ≤ 4 implies a well-differentiated tumour, 5–7 means a moderately differentiated cancer and > 7 is a poorly differentiated lesion.

38 CANCER GENETICS

A variety of hereditary conditions have now been extensively studied in the context of the development of colorectal cancer, and the genes responsible for tumour development continue to be elucidated. While such conditions are rare compared with sporadic tumours, representing only 5–10% of all such cancers, they are important not just for the families that have them (especially for screening and surveillance implications), but as an example of the increasing role of genomics and genetics in medicine and surgery.

1 C – Hereditary non-polyposis colorectal cancer (HNPCC)

These are the genetic defects classically associated with this condition in which affected individuals have a much greater than average chance of developing colorectal cancer. Compared with sporadic carcinomas, carcinomas develop at a younger age (typically in the 30–50-year age group), are often multiple (synchronous lesions), and are more commonly right-sided. The two commonest mutations are of the mismatch repair genes *MLH1* and *MSH2*, leading to DNA microsatellite instability. The condition is defined within families using the Amsterdam criteria (which can be remembered by 1,2,3):

- one case must be diagnosed before the age of 50 — 1
- one should be a first-degree relative of the other two — 1
- at least two successive generations should be affected — 2
- at least three relatives with colorectal cancer — 3

2 G – Peutz–Jeghers syndrome

The classical findings of this rare hereditary disorder are peri-oral and buccal mucosal pigmentation, multiple hamartomatous lesions throughout the gastrointestinal tract, particularly in the small intestine, and an increased risk of both intestinal and extra-intestinal malignancy. It is one of three clinically similar hamartomatous polyposis syndromes associated with colorectal cancer, the others being even rarer (Cowden's disease and juvenile polyposis). The mutant genes responsible have been elucidated for most cases.

3 E – *K-RAS* gene

K-RAS is located on chromosome 12 and plays a role in intracellular signal transduction. It is mutated in approximately 10% of adenomas that are < 1 cm, in 50% of adenomas > 1 cm, and in 50% of carcinomas. Other genetic abnormalities associated with colorectal cancer include inactivation of the *DCC* (Deleted in Colon Cancer) tumour suppressor gene that is located on chromosome 18 (18q21), mutation of the *APC* tumour suppressor gene on chromosome 5 (5q21) and loss of the *P53* gene on chromosome 17 (17p13.1).

39 COMMON CARCINOGENS

1 E – β-Naphthylamine

β-Naphthylamine is used in the paint and dye industry and is not intrinsically carcinogenic (a **remote** carcinogen), but it undergoes conjugation in the liver to create a water-soluble carcinogen (a **proximate** carcinogen). This conjugated carcinogen is excreted by the kidneys and stored in the bladder. Here, micro-organisms secrete glucuronidase, which releases the **ultimate** carcinogen into the bladder. This, over a period of exposure, can result in transitional cell carcinoma.

2 C – *Aspergillus flavus*

Aspergillus flavus produces Aflatoxin B1, which is a potent hepatocarcinogen in animals and is believed to be a factor in the high incidence of hepatocellular carcinoma in Africa (although you might not be blamed for choosing hepatitis B virus). *Aspergillus flavus* is a fungus that grows on grains and peanuts. Repeated ingestion of infected food is a risk factor.

3 Q – Schistosomiasis

This disease is caused by *Schistosoma haematobium*, a trematode fluke that lives in freshwater snails and parasitically in the human bladder. *Schistosoma* are found most commonly in Latin America, Africa and the Middle East. The eggs produced (up to hundreds a day) trigger granuloma formation which cause haematuria, cystitis, stenoses of the ureters and stone formation. The chronic inflammation induces squamous cell carcinoma of the bladder. Despite these urological manifestations, mortality is more commonly the result of portal vein granuloma formation with subsequent portal hypertension.

4 L – Human papillomavirus

Human papillomavirus (HPV) has been implicated as a promoter of cervical carcinoma; HPV types 6 and 11 predominate in lower grade dysplasias (cervical intraepithelial neoplasia – CIN 1), while higher-grade dysplasias (CIN 2 and CIN 3) tend to be associated with HPV types 16, 31 and 33. Other co-factors include infection with herpes simplex virus type 1 and tobacco use. The CIN stages represent carcinoma *in situ* and up to 70% of women in whom this is left untreated will progress to developing invasive cervical carcinoma.

SURGICAL SPECIALTIES

Cardiothoracic surgery

40 THORACIC TRAUMA

1 L – Tension pneumothorax

Initially the patient suffers an open pneumothorax ('sucking chest wound'), whereby the equilibrium between intrathoracic pressure and atmospheric pressure is immediate; if the defect is approximately two-thirds the tracheal width then the air follows the path of least resistance, through the defect, impairing ventilation. The paramedics were correct to close the defect; however, the dressing should only have been securely taped on three sides so as to create a flutter-type valve effect; this ensures the dressing is sucked over the defect on inspiration preventing air entering, while the open end allows air to escape on exhalation. By securing the dressing on all sides, air progressively accumulates in the thoracic cavity, collapsing the lung on the affected side. The mediastinum is displaced to the opposite side, decreasing venous return and compressing the opposite lung. The most common cause of tension pneumothorax is mechanical (positive-pressure) ventilation in the patient with a visceral pleural injury. Rapid decompression is required to prevent death.

2 G – Myocardial contusion

Blunt thoracic trauma can result in cardiac injury: myocardial muscle contusion, cardiac chamber rupture, or valvular disruption. Patients with myocardial contusion may complain of chest discomfort but this is often attributed to chest wall contusion or fractures of the sternum and/or ribs. The clinically important sequelae are hypotension, significant conduction abnormalities on electrocardiogram (ECG) or wall motion abnormality on two-dimensional echocardiography. Multiple premature ventricular contractions, unexplained sinus tachycardia, atrial fibrillation, bundle branch block (usually right), and ST segment changes are the most common ECG findings. Patients with myocardial contusion diagnosed by conduction abnormalities are at risk of sudden dysrhythmias and should be monitored for 24 h. After this time, the risk of sudden dysrhythmia substantially decreases.

3 J – Pulmonary contusion

Pulmonary contusion is the most common potentially lethal chest injury, commonly occurring secondary to multiple rib fractures or flail chest, as a result of blunt trauma. Respiratory failure may be subtle and develop over time as a result of underlying lung injury, rather than occur instantaneously. Patients with significant hypoxia (ie $p_A(O_2)$ < 8.0 kPa on room air, SaO_2 < 90%) and/or chronic lung disease will require intubation and ventilation.

41 CHEST TRAUMA MANAGEMENT

1 F – Insertion of chest drain

This patient probably has a haemothorax. The primary cause is either lung laceration or laceration of the intercostal/internal thoracic vessels. It is first treated with a large calibre chest drain [then intravenous access etc, following the ABC (Airways, Breathing, Circulation) protocol]. This not only evacuates the blood and reduces the risk of a clotted haemothorax, but also allows continuous monitoring of blood loss. Bleeding is usually self-limiting; however, if it continues, a thoracotomy may be required.

2 E – Immediate needle decompression

This lady has a tension pneumothorax, which develops when a 'one-way valve' air leak occurs either from the lung or through the chest wall. Air is forced into the thoracic cavity without means of escape, collapsing the affected lung. It is a clinical diagnosis and life-saving treatment, large-bore needle decompression into the second intercostal space in the mid-clavicular line of the affected hemithorax, should not be delayed by waiting for radiological confirmation. Clinical signs of tachypnoea, tachycardia, hypotension and neck vein distension may initially confuse diagnosis with cardiac tamponade. However, differentiation may be made by a hyper-resonant percussion note and/or the absence of breath sounds over the affected hemithorax.

3 H – Intubation and ventilation

This gentleman has a flail chest, which occurs when a segment of the chest wall loses bony continuity with the rest of the thoracic cage. It usually results from blunt trauma associated with multiple rib fractures. It is the underlying significant pulmonary contusion that is problematic. The definitive treatment is to re-expand the lung and ensure adequate oxygenation; in a hypoxic patient a short period of intubation and ventilation may be necessary until the diagnosis of the entire injury pattern is complete.

4 A – Arteriography

This gentleman has suffered traumatic aortic rupture. It is a common cause of death after a road traffic accident or after a fall from a great height. For immediate survivors, salvage is frequently possible if aortic rupture is identified and treated early. Patients with aortic rupture, who are potentially salvageable, tend to have a laceration near the ligamentum arteriosum. An intact adventitial layer or contained mediastinal haematoma prevents immediate death. Specific signs and symptoms are frequently absent. Its presence may be suggested by a characteristic widened mediastinum on chest X-ray. If aortic rupture is suspected, the patient should be evaluated by the most appropriate diagnostic tool determined by the doctors at the hospital at which the repair will be made. Angiography is considered the gold standard, although contrast computed tomography is often performed first.

5 J – Resuscitation (emergency room) thoracotomy

This is one of the two indications for this procedure (the other being massive tracheobronchial bleeding). In even relatively inexperienced hands, good results can be obtained if the cause is simple to address, eg myocardial puncture with tamponade. All other indications can probably wait until theatre where suitably trained staff are available (it is still termed an emergency thoracotomy, however). The method used to open the chest is a source of contention (the Editor prefers the clamshell approach).

42 LUNG CANCER: COMPLICATIONS

1 L – Pancoast's syndrome

This is a complication of an apically placed squamous cell carcinoma that invades directly into anatomical structures situated in this area including ribs, thoracic vertebrae and nerve roots. In addition to local symptoms, there are two resultant syndromes related to neuronal involvement. In this case, invasion of the brachial plexus roots leads to Pancoast's syndrome. The other well-recognised syndrome is Horner's syndrome, caused by involvement of sympathetic fibres as they exit the cord at T1 to ascend to the superior cervical ganglion (miosis, ptosis, enophthalmosis). NB Rather confusingly, a Pancoast tumour can lead to both Pancoast's and Horner's syndromes.

2 E – Ectopic antidiuretic hormone secretion (SIADH)

There are many causes for SIADH of which the paraneoplastic, ie non-metastatic, syndrome associated with small cell carcinoma of the lung is one. Inappropriate levels of the hormone lead to hypervolaemic hyponatraemia with inability of the body to diurese in response to falling plasma osmolality. Severe hyponatraemia with $Na^+ < 110$ mmol/litre can lead to generalised fits and coma.

3 K – Lambert–Eaton myasthenic syndrome (LEMS)

This is a rare, paraneoplastic syndrome associated with small cell carcinoma of the lung. There is impaired release of acetylcholine at the neuromuscular junction caused by autoantibodies directed to native calcium channels. The picture is therefore very similar to myasthenia gravis, typically with proximal weakness and often ocular or bulbar palsies. Unlike myasthenia gravis the weakness often improves with repeated muscle contraction. Other neural autoantibodies associated with small cell carcinoma include those to potassium channels leading to neuromyotonia (Isaac's syndrome) and those leading to cerebellar ataxia and other peripheral neuropathies.

General surgery

43 COMMON ABDOMINAL OPERATIONS

1 D – Hartmann's procedure

The clinical picture is that of a perforated diverticulum with faecal peritonitis. In an elderly patient with gross faecal peritonitis the mortality rate is over 50% and in such circumstances a lengthy procedure is not indicated. In selected cases with a small leak, minimal soiling and a fit patient, primary resection with on-table lavage and anastomosis can be performed. However, this is not indicated in the case described. Hartmann's procedure is also used in an emergency for obstructing conditions affecting the sigmoid region of the colon (especially in high-risk patients). The diseased or obstructed area is excised but an anastomosis of the bowel is not undertaken for reasons of safety at the time, and the high risk of anastomotic dehiscence post-operatively. The proximal colon is therefore brought to the skin as a stoma and the rectal stump is oversewn. The colostomy may be reversed at a later date, but this in itself is no small undertaking.

2 J – Right hemicolectomy

Surgical resection will not cure Crohn's disease and is usually performed for complications. The overall strategy is to be as conservative as possible to preserve functional gut length. Indications for surgery include recurrent intestinal obstruction, intestinal fistulae, fulminant colitis, malignant change and peri-anal disease. The whole of the gastrointestinal tract should be examined prior to undertaking any resection either pre-operatively or at laparotomy. In this particular case, a right hemicolectomy is the operation of choice as the patient will probably have isolated terminal ileal disease. Proximal small bowel strictures can be treated with segmental resection if only isolated areas are affected, or alternatively, with stricturoplasty of multiple involved segments.

3 L – Total mesorectal excision (TME)

This is the operation of choice for middle and lower third tumours of the rectum that are amenable to resection without recourse to abdomino-perineal excision of rectum (APER). The operation, championed by Bill Heald, attends to the main cause of local failure (recurrence) of cancer by addressing both the circumferential resection margins as well as the distal resection margin. APER is used when an adequate distal resection margin is not achievable by abdominal approach – usually because the tumour has invaded the sphincters.

44 HERNIAS (TYPES AND TAXONOMY)

1 H – Maydl's hernia

Maydl's hernia is a complication of large hernial sacs, especially right scrotal hernias in Africans. It is characterised by a W-loop of small bowel lying in the sac, with strangulation of the 'intervening' loop within the main abdominal cavity by the constriction of the neck of the sac. The description of the operative findings differentiates this hernia from afferent loop strangulation (afferent loop entwined about afferent and efferent loops), a Richter's hernia (part of the bowel at the anti-mesenteric margin becomes strangulated), and a Littre's hernia (strangulation of a Meckel's diverticulum). The operative findings also differentiate from 'simple' strangulation, which is associated with a similar clinical presentation, ie evidence of gut ischaemia (severe pain with systemic upset, eg fever, tachycardia) and obstruction (vomiting, and abdominal pain and distension).

2 J – Obturator hernia

Obturator hernias are six times more common in women than men, and three times more common after than before the age of 50 years. A pre-operative diagnosis is rarely made, because a swelling is not always palpable in the thigh. Therefore, it is usually diagnosed during laparotomy for non-resolving small bowel obstruction, as in the case described. Consequently, the operative mortality is approximately 30%. The peritoneum protrudes through the obturator canal, and then between the pectineus and abductor longus muscles to enter the femoral triangle. The Howship–Romberg sign of pain referred along the geniculate branch of the obturator nerve to the inner aspect of the knee should raise the suspicion of an obturator hernia. Other examples of hernias frequently only discovered during laparotomy for relief of intestinal obstruction include: gluteal and sciatic hernias (protruding through the greater and lesser sciatic notches, respectively), pelvic hernias (of the pouch of Douglas into the posterior wall of the vagina or vulva; not rectocoele or cystocoele, which are false hernias), and pudendal hernias (lateral protrusion of peritoneum through a persistent hiatus of Schwalbe between the origin of the levator ani from the obturator internus, usually following surgical removal of pelvic organs).

3 C – Incarcerated hernia

This question draws the candidates' attention to the clinical differentiation of complications of hernias. Incarceration refers to fixation of contents within the hernia sac as a result of adhesions. Such a hernia is irreducible, but is neither tender, nor associated with systemic upset (differentiating it from a strangulated hernia), nor associated with gastrointestinal symptoms (differentiating it from an obstructed hernia).

45 MANAGEMENT OF GROIN HERNIAS

1 H – McEvedie's approach (or modification)

The patient has an obstructed, strangulated femoral hernia. There are three approaches to femoral hernia repair and although opinion varies, the safest surgical approach (after resuscitation) in this patient (with the expectation of bowel injury and resection) is a modified McEvedie using an incision resembling half of a Pfannenstiel incision (the original McEvedie had a vertical incision necessitating division of the inguinal ligament). The pre-peritoneal space is tracked downwards and the hernia is opened. If a bowel resection is required a laparotomy can easily be performed either through this incision or by its extension to a full Pfannenstiel. If strangulation was not expected then the low crural approach (basically a small incision over the lump) is preferred. The high crural approach disrupts the posterior wall of the inguinal canal and has fallen from favour (in some textbooks).

2 E – Lichtenstein repair

Based on relative ease of procedure and low recurrence rate, this repair using a polypropelene mesh is now recommended (including by the Royal College of Surgeons) as the mainstay of primary hernia repair (replacing Shouldice which was probably slightly more complex to perform adequately in most hands but still has its proponents). The recurrence rate should be < 1%. Discussion continues regarding laparoscopic approaches (listed). NICE recommends laparoscopic hernia repair for recurrent and bilateral hernia. A recent randomised controlled trial in the *New England Journal* (2004) suggests a higher recurrence rate when used for primary hernia compared with current open approaches. The Bassini repair is outdated (pain, recurrence etc).

3 B – Herniogram

This is the investigation of choice when no lump is evident. In contrast, if a lump had been present but you were unconvinced that this was a hernia then an ultrasound to distinguish the lump would be the preferred investigation.

4 C – Herniotomy

Herniorrhaphies, ie repair of the retaining wall, are not required for infantile/childhood inguinal hernias where the cause is patency of the processus vaginalis. The sac is identified and carefully dissected from the cord, its contents are emptied and the sac is then ligated and excised. This should be delayed (but only briefly) if the incarceration can be managed initially conservatively as in this case.

46 GROIN LUMPS

1 I – Psoas abscess

Although this mass could be attributed to lymphadenopathy (probably secondary to his clear history of tuberculosis), the fluctuant nature and the presence of ipsilateral hip pain point more readily to symptoms of a psoas abscess. Psoas abscesses develop either from infection of unknown origin or as a consequence of infection spreading from an adjacent organ. The risk factors for primary psoas abscess are not known; however, trauma to the muscle may be an important factor in 18–20% of cases. Low socio-economic class and poor nutrition have also been cited as possible predisposing factors. A major risk factor for secondary psoas abscess is gastrointestinal pathology (inflammatory bowel disease, appendicitis, diverticulitis, bowel cancer and Crohn's disease), and the source is a gastro-intestinal infection in 80% of individuals. Prior to modern anti-tuberculous therapy, psoas abscesses occurred in up to 20% of patients with spinal tuberculosis. Treatment is now usually (initially at least) by percutaneous drainage under ultrasound or computed tomography guidance.

2 C – Femoral hernia

This gentleman has signs of small bowel obstruction secondary to a strangulated femoral hernia. A small complicated hernia present in the groin crease in the elderly with no prior history of a reducible lump is much more likely to be a femoral than an inguinal hernia (although inguinal hernias are approximately ten times more common in general).

3 H – Pseudo-aneurysm

The nature of this man's investigation points to the diagnosis of a pseudo-aneurysm. Failure to compress the site of arterial cannulation (a traumatic breach to the vessel wall) leads to extravasation of arterial blood. A haematoma then forms in the soft tissues around the artery, which produces a transmissible pulse. A true aneurysm is one that involves all the layers of the arterial wall (three layers) and is described as being expansile.

47 RIGHT ILIAC FOSSA MASS

Note: The candidate can approach the differentiation of right iliac fossa masses by remembering the few common causes or alternatively by taking a systematic anatomical approach, starting at the anterior abdominal wall and moving back towards the retroperitoneum (see right iliac fossa pain).

1 C – Appendix mass

The natural history of untreated acute appendicitis is that it will resolve, become gangrenous and perforate, or it will become surrounded by a mass of omentum and small bowel that walls off the inflammatory process and prevents inflammatory spread to the abdominal cavity yet delays resolution of the condition. Such patients usually present with a longer history (a week or more) of right lower quadrant abdominal pain. On examination the patient has a persistent low-grade fever, mild tachycardia and there is a tender indistinct mass in the right iliac fossa. The condition is usually best managed conservatively, as the risk of perforation has passed and removal of the appendix can be difficult. This differs from appendix abscess, when a perforated appendix becomes walled off by omentum. Unlike an appendix mass, the patient with an appendix abscess becomes systemically unwell with intermittent swinging pyrexia, rigors and profuse sweating. Drainage, either under radiological control or surgically, is the best initial treatment.

2 E – Crohn's disease

The long-standing history of typical symptoms should alert you to this diagnosis. Examination findings often only reveal right lower quadrant tenderness; however, a mass can sometimes be felt secondary to thickened or matted loops of inflamed bowel plus localised perforation with fistulation/interloop abscess.

3 D – Caecal carcinoma

This needs to be excluded in any patient presenting in their sixth to eighth decade with anaemia, unexplained weight loss, or abdominal pain.

48 THE ACUTE ABDOMEN: INVESTIGATION AND MANAGEMENT

1 B – Computed tomography (CT) scan

The clinical findings, taken together with this gentleman's associated risk factors, strongly suggest a diagnosis of dissecting abdominal aneurysm. The first step in investigation is a contrast CT scan to establish the diagnosis and extent of the problem and so plan surgical or endoprosthetic management.

2 E – Laparotomy

This woman is suffering from large bowel obstruction. The right iliac fossa peritonism is secondary to caecal distension and wall ischaemia. Laparotomy should not be delayed beyond resuscitation in this instance because caecal perforation with faecal peritonitis is imminent (and usually fatal). Note (see question 59 on large bowel obstruction) that when such signs are not present, further investigation to exclude pseudo-obstruction should be performed (water-soluble contrast enema or contrast CT).

3 C – Diagnostic laparoscopy

This young woman's symptoms may be caused by an underlying appendicitis or related to a recurrence of her ovarian cystic pathology. Ovarian cysts may tort and infarct or rupture, producing severe abdominal pain and low-grade fever that can closely mimic the signs and symptoms of appendicitis. In the face of uncertainty, a diagnostic laparoscopy would be most appropriate to allow the management of either pathology. Its use is associated with a reduction in the rate of negative appendicectomy and can also be used in the diagnosis of other causes of peritonitis.

4 B – CT scan

This is a challenging but not uncommon presentation. You cannot clinically differentiate between acute on chronic pancreatitis with a normal amylase and a perforated duodenal ulcer with no free gas (50% do not). Rather than performing a laparotomy, a CT scan is appropriate, principally because of its high sensitivity of picking up free gas/fluid.

49 THE ACUTE ABDOMEN

The term 'the acute abdomen' describes a non-traumatic event affecting any of the abdominal organs following which the characteristic, common presenting feature is severe abdominal pain. Exactly where one places the cut-off in terms of severity is probably arguable with some (the majority) placing most acute abdominal inflammatory and obstructive processes under the umbrella (as above) and others reserving the term for the catastrophe, eg perforations/haemorrhage/ischaemia.

1 J – Mesenteric infarction

This woman's irregular heart rhythm has provided the right environment for clot (think of Virchow's triad) and subsequent embolus formation. Emboli can lodge anywhere in the systemic circulation including the mesenteric arteries. An acute embolus blocking the origin of the superior mesenteric artery with propagating thrombus extending into smaller vessels usually produces mesenteric ischaemia. It can be notoriously difficult to diagnose but should be suspected especially when pain is out of proportion to evident clinical signs as in this case. A full classification is:

Occlusive

- mesenteric embolus, eg from the left atrium in atrial fibrillation
- mesenteric arterial thrombosis secondary to atheroma
- mesenteric venous occlusion, eg portal hypertension, and

Non-occlusive

- occurs in patients with a grossly diminished cardiac output, eg following myocardial infarction.

2 E – Diverticulitis

This is without doubt the commonest cause of acute left iliac fossa pain and peritonism in this age group.

3 N – Ureteric colic

The history of sudden onset of severe colic indicates that you are dealing with a luminal obstruction not an inflammatory cause. In a man of this age, ureteric colic is top of the list. The diagnosis is strongly supported by blood in the urine. An intravenous urogram or computed tomographic study of the kidney and upper bladder can be used to confirm the diagnosis.

50 EPIGASTRIC PAIN/DYSPEPSIA: MANAGEMENT

1 K – Proton pump inhibitor

The endoscopic findings are consistent with a diagnosis of gastro-oesophageal reflux disease. Having made the diagnosis, treatment is via a reduction in exacerbating factors such as smoking and alcohol, and the administration of antacids and importantly proton pump inhibitors. Refractory cases may be candidates for laparoscopic Nissen's fundoplication.

2 D – Emergency laparotomy

Uncontrollable bleeding at endoscopy is one of the indications for surgery in upper gastrointestinal haemorrhage. Other indications (in most units) include:

- patient > 55 years with three bleeds or more
- patient > 60 years with two or more bleeds
- transfusion requirement of six or more units
- visible arterial spurter in base of ulcer at endoscopy.

3 C – Computed tomography scan – chest and abdomen

The endoscopic findings suggest a diagnosis of adenocarcinoma of the oesophagus. In the case of tumours of the lower third, spread is local (to the adjacent organs), lymphatic (to the gastric and coeliac nodes) and haematogenous (to the liver). In all patients, a computed tomography scan of the chest and abdomen aids in staging the disease.

4 J – Prokinetic drug

The patient has gastroparesis, a complication occurring in up to 20% of patients with type I diabetes (insulin-dependent diabetes mellitus) and less often in type II disease. Gastroparesis probably occurs as a result of vagal neuropathy. Symptoms include: vomiting, early satiety, bloating, pain and weight loss. Endoscopic findings are similar to those found in pyloric stenosis, ie a large stomach full of food. The crucial difference is that no obstructing lesion or stricture is found. Treatment is by prokinetic drugs such as metoclopramide or erythromycin. Some research suggests a role for laparoscopic gastric pacing.

51 RIGHT ILIAC FOSSA PAIN (COMMON CAUSES)

It is easily possible to name at least 20 causes of right iliac fossa pain. The list given in this question includes some of the more common ones. In general, like so much of medicine, it is more common to see a common condition presenting atypically than a rare condition presenting typically, eg a urinary tract infection while usually associated with suprapubic pain may also present with right iliac fossa pain. For a complete list consider the contents of abdomen anatomically from front to back in the region of the right iliac fossa. Hence, (1) anterior abdominal wall, eg rectus sheath haematoma, (2) peritoneal viscera: caecum, small intestine, appendix, right fallopian tube and ovary, bladder, (3) retroperitoneal structures: kidney, ureter, iliac artery (leaking aneurysm thereof), undescended testis (torsion thereof), psoas muscle (abscess). The two commonest final diagnoses are non-specific abdominal pain and appendicitis.

1 A – Acute appendicitis
This should be obvious.

2 F – Irritable bowel syndrome
This 'non-diagnosis' is suggested by the long history and typical symptoms fulfilling the Rome criteria that are based on the clustering of certain symptoms in population studies (now defined by Rome II criteria). Clearly, irritable bowel syndrome should only be diagnosed when an organic cause for the patient's symptoms has been excluded. Patients are typically young or middle-aged women, as in this case.

3 J – Ruptured ectopic pregnancy
'Every woman of child-bearing age is pregnant until proven otherwise.' The typical history is of abdominal pain associated with fainting or collapse. Symptoms and signs of shock are usually present and, in the case of intraperitoneal rupture, diaphragmatic irritation gives referred pain to the shoulder. There may be a history of a missed menstrual period, but symptoms of tubal pregnancy may occur before this occurs. It is unusual for a tubal pregnancy to advance beyond 6–8 weeks without symptoms. There is usually a degree of abdominal distension and sub-umbilical tenderness and guarding. A urinary or serum β-human chorionic gonadotrophin measurement aids in the diagnosis. Prompt treatment is important and includes resuscitation followed by urgent laparoscopy or laparotomy depending on the availability of trained staff.

4 K – Torsion ovarian cyst

The history of sudden onset of pain without gastrointestinal disturbance suggests this diagnosis, which is a common differential in young women. The diagnosis can usually be confirmed by pelvic or transvaginal ultrasound examination, and commonly requires surgery. A similar presentation is seen with haemorrhage into and rupture of an ovarian cyst.

52 RIGHT ILIAC FOSSA PAIN (RARE CAUSES)

1 H – Rectus sheath haematoma

This occurs following rupture of the inferior epigastric artery, typically after coughing or straining. The site of the haematoma is usually at the level of the arcuate line and produces a mass in the relevant iliac fossa. The lump is related to the muscles of the anterior abdominal wall, contraction of which makes the lump indistinct. Bruising may not always be apparent. The condition occurs in three distinct groups of individuals: elderly women, pregnant women and athletic, muscular men. Exploration of the anterior abdominal wall, evacuation of haematoma and ligation of the bleeding vessel may be required, however, small haematomas can be treated conservatively.

2 G – Psoas abscess

The history of a long period of ill health and backache is highly suggestive of spinal tuberculosis, the commonest site of skeletal disease. Caseation and cold abscess formation extends into the paravertebral soft tissues with the formation of a psoas abscess, which may point to the groin. There is a risk of cord compression from vertebral collapse or pressure from the abscess. Treatment is with anti-tuberculosis chemotherapy, with surgery reserved for drainage of abscesses, skeletal deformity and cord compression.

53 CHRONIC NON-MALIGNANT PELVIC PAIN IN WOMEN

There are numerous causes of chronic non-malignant pelvic pain in women. For convenience, they may be classified anatomically according to the contents of the pelvis, ie lower urinary tract disorders, disorders of the reproductive organs, gastrointestinal disorders. In addition, it is important to consider that pain may be musculo-skeletal, neurogenic, or psychological in origin. Accordingly, the list of causes provided in the question may be classified to produce a differential diagnosis for chronic pelvic pain that incorporates the commonest causes for each 'system'. The surgical trainee should be alert to causes originating 'outside' the gastro-intestinal system, so that patients may be referred to the appropriate specialist for further assessment.

1 O – Utero-vaginal prolapse

Utero-vaginal prolapse is related to pelvic floor trauma sustained during childbirth and oestrogen deficiency following the menopause. Typically, symptoms associated with genital prolapse include a dragging sensation in the pelvis or awareness of 'something coming down'. Resultant pelvic floor dysfunction impacts on urinary, sexual and rectal evacuatory function, resulting in voiding difficulties/urinary incontinence, impaired coitus and evacuation difficulties, respectively. The multi-system disruption of pelvic organ function suggests the diagnosis, which is confirmed on clinical examination. Such patients are prone to bladder and rectal prolapse as a result of weakening of the pelvic floor musculature. Treatment may include non-surgical measures (pelvic floor physiotherapy, oestrogen replacement therapy and intravaginal devices), although surgery to eliminate the prolapse and restore pelvic floor function offers definitive treatment.

2 A – Benign ovarian tumour

Benign ovarian tumours are common in this age group. Most tumours of the ovary are simply large versions of the cysts that form during the normal ovarian cycle, and so are small, asymptomatic and resolve spontaneously. These are termed 'functional' cysts. Benign germ cell tumours (eg dermoid cyst) are also common in women less than 30 years of age. Other histological types include benign epithelial and sex cord stromal tumours. Symptoms tend not to occur until the tumour is larger than 3–5 cm, although complications such as rupture, haemorrhage, or infection may result in acute pelvic pain. Occasionally, large tumours may give rise to urinary or gastrointestinal symptoms because of pressure effects. Menstrual disturbance is uncommon, unless the tumour secretes oestrogens (sex cord tumours). Cyst formation may complicate endometriosis (endometrioma), but here the clinical picture is usually of dysmenorrhoea, dyspareunia and sub-fertility.

3 I – Painful bladder syndrome

Patients with painful bladder syndrome complain of bladder pain and irritative bladder symptoms (frequency, urgency, nocturia and dysuria). The bladder pain is worse when the bladder is distended, and often improved following micturition. Urine cultures are repeatedly negative, leading the unwary to exclude a urinary cause of pain in such patients. Causes include radiation, chemical and interstitial cystitis. Urine should be cultured for atypical organisms (*Mycoplasma* and *Ureaplasma*). Cystometry and cystoscopy are useful diagnostic tests and often reveal a low capacity, non-compliant ('stiff') bladder. Cystoscopy may reveal subepithelial haemorrhages in patients with interstitial cystitis and allows biopsies to be taken for histological confirmation of this condition.

4 E – Diverticular disease

Patients with diverticular disease commonly complain of episodic lower abdominal pain, although some authorities question the existence of painful diverticular disease. The pain may be associated with a change in bowel habit and abdominal bloating, making clinical differentiation from irritable bowel syndrome difficult. A positive history of brisk bleeding per rectum supports a diagnosis of diverticular disease, because haemorrhage is another of the complications of this disease. The history is not that of inflammatory bowel disease.

54 THE ABDOMINAL MASS

1 C – Carcinoma of the caecum

In contrast with left-sided tumours, caecal carcinoma has an insidious onset with generalised features of malignant disease, such as anaemia, anorexia, weight loss and lethargy. Late features include a palpable mass in the right iliac fossa and obstruction to the ileocaecal valve resulting in small bowel obstruction. Obstruction of the appendiceal orifice can give rise to symptoms and signs of acute appendicitis, a fact that should be remembered when faced with a patient over the age of 40 with appendicitis.

2 D – Carcinoma of the head of the pancreas

The history and findings are of obstructive jaundice with a palpable gallbladder. Courvoisier's law states 'when the gallbladder is palpable and the patient is jaundiced, the obstruction of the bile duct causing the jaundice is unlikely to be a stone because previous inflammation will have made the gallbladder thick and non-distensible'. While there are a few exceptions to this rule, the history of substantial weight loss, and of pain radiating to the left side of the back strongly indicate the likelihood of pancreatic carcinoma – which is the commonest cause of malignant biliary obstruction.

3 K – Mesenteric cyst

These cysts are found most commonly in the mesentery of the ileum arising from congenitally misplaced lymphatic tissue (chylolymphatic cyst) or from remnants of reduplicated bowel (enterogenous cyst). They typically present in the second decade of life as a painless swelling or with recurrent episodes of abdominal pain. Acute abdominal pain may arise following rupture or bleeding into a cyst. On examination the characteristic finding is that of a fluctuant, resonant, spherical swelling, close to the umbilicus. The cyst is freely mobile in a plane at right angles to the root of the mesentery and may 'slip' during the course of the examination.

55 HEPATOMEGALY

1 O – Riedel's lobe

This scenario describes the congenital anomaly of a Riedel's lobe. This is a projection of normally functioning liver tissue downward from the right lobe of the liver, below the costal margin and along the anterior axillary line. It can be mistaken for a pathological enlargement of the liver or the gallbladder, but is a normal anatomical variation (hence the unremarkable liver function tests).

2 F – Hepatocellular carcinoma

Hepatocellular carcinoma is one of the most common cancers world-wide, although it is rarer in the Western world. It accounts for 90% of primary hepatic malignancies and is endemic in regions where hepatitis is rife. In this particular case, it is probably associated with chronic hepatitis contracted from a contaminated blood transfusion. It should be suspected in any patient in whom liver function rapidly deteriorates on a background of known hepatitis or cirrhosis.

56 CONDITIONS THAT MAY REQUIRE SPLENECTOMY

There are a myriad of causes of splenomegaly which the 'diagnostic sieve' approach can usually resolve. The list above includes some of the more common faced by the surgeon for consideration of splenectomy. The main indication outside trauma (blunt or iatrogenic) for splenectomy is 'hyper-splenism', which is a rather indefinite syndrome characterised by enlargement, and any combination of anaemia, leukopenia and thrombo-cytopaenia, bone marrow hyperplasia and improvement after splenectomy.

1 C – Congenital spherocytosis

Approximately 75% of cases are autosomal dominant disorders characterised by defects in the red cell membrane that render erythrocytes spheroidal, less deformable and vulnerable to splenic sequestration. Anaemia, moderate splenomegaly and jaundice are characteristic. After 10 years of age, 40–50% of patients develop gallstones secondary to hyperbilirubinaemia. Splenectomy is indicated in the majority of patients, as red cell survival reverts to normal even though the abnormality persists.

2 B – Chronic myeloid leukaemia

This primarily affects adults in the 4th and 5th decades of life, accounting for 15–20% of all cases of leukaemia. It is a clonal disorder of pluripotent stem cells that predominantly differentiate along the granulocytic pathway. Initial symptoms are non-specific; however, a dragging sensation in the abdomen caused by extreme splenomegaly is characteristic. Symptomatic hypersplenism may occur during the chronic phase of the disorder and may require splenectomy.

3 J – Splenic abscess

Splenic abscesses are rare, probably because of the spleen's exceptional ability to cope with septic and foreign material. They may, however occur as a result of haematogenous spread as in this case with the clinical triad of left upper quadrant pain, fever and systemic signs of sepsis. Treatment is usually by percutaneous drainage of the abscess and treatment of the cause.

57 COMPLICATIONS OF SPLENECTOMY

Some operations have a good list of specific complications that are beloved of examiners. Favoured are probably thyroidectomy, splenectomy, laparoscopic cholecystectomy and inguinal hernia repair.

1 F – Overwhelming post-splenectomy sepsis

After splenectomy the ability of the spleen to destroy encapsulated organisms is lost and infection can lead to the distinct clinical syndrome of overwhelming post-splenectomy infection (OPSI). In children splenectomised for trauma the incidence is about 1–2%, while for adults it is about 0.5%. Long-term penicillins are of proven value in children, as the maximal incidence of OPSI occurs within 2 years of surgery. Prophylaxis with polyvalent vaccines is also recommended (usually to pneumococcus, meningococcus and *Haemophilus influenzae*).

2 L – Subphrenic abscess

Post-operative haematomas are common post-splenectomy. They may collect in the subphrenic space, and infection can readily lead to a subphrenic abscess. They may cause an associated pleural effusion as in this case. Characteristically they present with swinging pyrexia, sweats, rigors and left-sided pain on deep inspiration. Treatment is usually by percutaneous drainage.

58 INTESTINAL OBSTRUCTION

1 H – Gallstone ileus

Gallstones are responsible for less than 1% of all cases of small bowel obstruction. About 90% of stones entering the intestine will impact in the terminal ileum, although other reported sites include the duodenum, jejunum, colon and rectum. A stone formed in the gall bladder enters the small bowel via a biliary-enteric fistula, usually between the gallbladder and duodenum. Patients tend to be elderly and often do not report a history of cholecystitis. On X-ray the presence of a pneumobilia is pathognomic, provided there is no recent history of biliary-intestinal bypass or sphincterotomy.

2 M – Volvulus

The case gives the classical history of a patient with a sigmoid volvulus who is typically elderly and institutionalised, suffering with chronic constipation and regular laxative use. There is usually a history of similar episodes in the past, which resolve following 'untwisting of the sigmoid mesentery'. Typical X-ray findings are of a large oval gas shadow on the left hand side, which is looped onto itself, the so-called 'bent inner tube' or 'coffee bean' sign. Treatment is by decompression by means of a flatus tube inserted via a sigmoidoscope, done of course at arm's length! Should this fail then operative 'untwisting' with or without resection may be required.

3 D – Crohn's disease

The history is fairly typical of that for ileocaecal Crohn's disease (the commonest site: 50%). Disease of the terminal ileum may result in fine string-like-calibre strictures in the right iliac fossa on barium studies. This is known as the 'string sign of Kantor'.

4 K – Intestinal pseudo-obstruction

This is a bit of an honours question – it is one of the rarer paraneoplastic syndromes associated with small cell carcinoma. It is caused by an autoimmune inflammation/destruction of the myenteric plexus.

59 LARGE BOWEL OBSTRUCTION

There are four common causes of large bowel obstruction in Western society: carcinoma, diverticular disease, volvulus (principally sigmoid) and pseudo-obstruction.

1 D – Diverticular disease

The diagnosis is suggested by the long history of constipation and recurrent abdominal pain in an otherwise fit and well elderly woman. Inflammation of one or more diverticula may result in haemorrhage, perforation, or resolution with fibrosis. Repeated episodes of inflammation can give rise to the formation of a fibrotic, inflammatory stricture with symptoms and signs of bowel obstruction. This may be acute, chronic, or acute on chronic. In many cases the clinical picture can be difficult to differentiate from colonic carcinoma and a definitive diagnosis may not be possible until histological examination of specimens resected at laparotomy is done.

2 J – Pseudo-obstruction

In a large hospital, barely a week goes by without being referred such a patient either by the medical, neurosurgical, or orthopaedic teams. Colonic pseudo-obstruction probably represents about a quarter of all large bowel obstruction. It is a reactive dilatation and ileus, presumed (although not-proven) to be secondary to disturbed autonomic (cholinergic) innervation. Classic conditions that may precipitate it are sepsis, especially chest infections, cerebrovascular accident/neurosurgery, fractured NOF, and spinal/retroperitoneal surgery (these probably directly disrupt nerves – indeed, the condition was first described in this respect with retroperitoneal tumours (Ogilvie's syndrome).

3 H – Ischaemic stricture

Ischaemia of the left hemicolon is a recognised complication of abdominal aortic aneurysm repair and occurs as a result of an insufficient collateral blood supply from the marginal artery following ligation of the inferior mesenteric artery. Presentation may be acute, with the passage of bloody diarrhoea, or insidious as in the case described. The region of the splenic flexure is commonly affected and chronic ischaemia may result in the formation of a stricture, indistinguishable from a carcinoma on barium enema examination. Mesenteric arteriography confirms the diagnosis.

60 ABDOMINAL DISTENSION

The list includes some of the principal causes of abdominal distension. These can be more easily remembered by the five 'F's – Flatus, Faeces, Fluid, Fetus and Fantastically large organs and tumours.

1 I – Ovarian cyst/tumour

The patient has a large cystic swelling arising from the pelvis, as evidenced by the clinical findings of an indistinct lower border (unable to get below it on clinical examination) and a resonant percussion note. The differential diagnosis is an ovarian cyst or urinary bladder. However, chronic retention of urine in women is uncommon and unlikely to cause enlargement to this degree. Ovarian cysts may be of any size and on occasion can reach enormous proportions. These tend to be of the benign mucinous variety. Large cysts may press on the bladder, reducing its volume and causing increased frequency of micturition. The effects of a large space-occupying lesion in the abdomen may also cause respiratory embarrassment. Ultrasound scanning is useful as it not only confirms the diagnosis, but also provides a clue as to the nature; true cystic lesions without solid elements are rarely malignant.

2 M – Retroperitoneal sarcoma

Retroperitoneal tumours can grow to enormous proportions with patients presenting on account of abdominal distension, vague abdominal pain, or general features of malignant disease. The mass may result in ureteric obstruction or displacement and may give rise to features of bowel obstruction through pressure on the colon. On examination these tumours are indistinguishable from an enlarged kidney and require computed tomography scanning for differentiation between the two.

3 G – Massive splenomegaly

The patient has features of falciparum malaria, which typically gives rise to a prodromal illness of malaise, myalgia, headaches and anorexia, followed by paroxysms of sweating, fever and rigors. The abdominal distension is the result of massive splenomegaly, the main causes of which are listed below:

- chronic myeloid leukaemia
- myelofibrosis
- leishmaniasis
- schistosomiasis
- malaria
- tropical splenomegaly.

61 DYSPHAGIA

1 E – Diffuse oesophageal spasm

This is a clinical syndrome characterised by symptoms of retrosternal chest pain and/or intermittent dysphagia. The chest pain can be severe and is frequently mistaken as cardiac in origin. Initially described by Osgood in 1889, the first manometric descriptions were not until 1958. Before manometry, the diagnosis relied on the symptom complex and the radiological findings of a normal oesophageal lumen, failure of peristaltic propagation, and simultaneous oesophageal contractions, sometimes resulting in a beaded appearance. A variety of radiological appearances and terminologies have been used such as 'pseudodiverticulosis', 'segmental spasms', and 'corkscrew oesophagus', although in most cases the diagnosis would be missed by barium swallow/gastroscopy as the oesophagus usually appears normal.

2 B – Bulbar palsy

This is a palsy of the tongue, muscles of mastication, muscles of deglutition, and facial muscles as a result of loss of function of brainstem motor nuclei. The signs are those of a lower motor neurone lesion. Bulbar palsy is one of the principal clinical patterns distinguished in motor neurone disease (MND) (25% of cases); other causes include Guillain–Barré syndrome, polio and brainstem tumours. MND never affects the extraocular movements, distinguishing it from myasthenia gravis. In contrast to bulbar palsy, pseudobulbar palsy is an upper motor neurone lesion usually caused by stroke.

3 J – Oesophageal carcinoma

While this might be deemed a slightly unfair question, the history of rapidly progressive dysphagia in a man of this age (despite his nationality) should prompt this diagnosis rather than that of Chagas' disease. The latter disorder is caused by the parasite *Trypanosoma cruzi* and is endemic in large parts of rural South America (including Brazil), making it one of the commonest diseases in the world. However, the complication of megaoesophagus is relatively uncommon (25% cases) compared with the main manifestation (cardiomyopathy). In addition, the oesophageal manifestations are similar to achalasia clinically, ie a non-progressive dysphagia to liquids (as well as pathologically: destruction of the myenteric plexus).

62 VOMITING

*It is not impossible to list approximately 150 causes of nausea and vomiting. Broadly, however, a complete overview of **all** the causes of vomiting includes five groups:*

- *central (intracranial, labyrinthine etc)*
- *metabolic and endocrine (uraemia, pregnancy, diabetes etc)*
- *iatrogenic (cancer chemotherapy, digoxin, opiates etc)*
- *obstructive (any level), and*
- *mucosal inflammation (appendicitis, gastritis, cholecystitis etc).*

1 E – Gastritis

This, and enteritis, are probably the commonest causes of vomiting seen in a typical Emergency Department. Enteritis tends to have little in the way of epigastric pain and more central colic with or without diarrhoea.

2 A – Drug-related

This lady has post-operative nausea and vomiting (PONV). The problem is multifactorial but is principally related to anaesthetic drugs. It is three times more common in women and is best prevented rather than treated.

63 INVESTIGATION AND MANAGEMENT OF GASTROINTESTINAL BLEEDING

1 H – OGD and adrenaline injection

In such a situation it is recommended that haemostasis is attempted with injection of 1 : 10, 000 adrenaline. Although evidence-based practice has shown heat probe, bipolar diathermy and injection sclerotherapy all to be effective, adrenaline injection is often used in combination with these modalities, and available trials show that adrenaline alone is equally effective. Repeated injection of fibrin glue or the application of micro-clips should be limited to specialist centres where operators are undertaking such procedures on a regular basis, and hence have special expertise. Only if this fails or if there are other endoscopic or clinical indications should the patient undergo surgery (under-running of ulcer).

2 L – Proctosigmoidoscopy

This is the first investigation of choice and will yield the cause (piles) in many cases, both in outpatients and The Emergency Department. If no evident cause is found in the anorectum and fresh bleeding continues, a flexible sigmoidoscopy would be the next step. In contrast, dark-red bleeding/melaena, or associated change in bowel habit to loose stool/diarrhoea would favour a full colonoscopy.

3 A – Angiography

Despite aggressive resuscitation, this woman appears to have an unrelenting small bowel/proximal colonic haemorrhage (melaena plus dark fresh blood). Although ultimately she is likely to require a laparotomy, the intermediate step is to undertake an emergency mesenteric angiogram in an attempt to discover the origin of the bleed. This can localise bleeding in 58–86% of patients who have active bleeding (classified as a rate of 1–1.5 ml/min). Positive angiography may allow immediate therapeutic intervention via embolisation with metal microcoils or gelfoams. In addition, intra-arterial vasopressin at angiography has a good initial haemostatic capability; however the rate of re-bleeding is high. Clearly if these attempts fail (either to localise or control the haemorrhage) an emergency laparotomy, with on-table endoscopy/enteroscopy, should be performed.

64 HAEMATEMESIS

1 D – Duodenal ulcer

The history of recent non-steroidal anti-inflammatory drug (NSAID) use, on a chronic background of dyspeptic symptoms, with the vomiting of altered blood, points to either peptic ulcer disease or erosive gastritis. However, epigastric pain that is relieved by eating is said to be commonly experienced by those suffering from duodenal ulcer. Other features that are more predictive of duodenal ulcer disease include pain that worsens when the patient is experiencing stress and anxiety, and the presence of nocturnal dyspepsia. Investigation should be by gastroscopy with or without endoscopic therapy if actively bleeding (emergency not required in this case). Management involves cessation of NSAIDs and continued medical therapy with histamine antagonists or proton pump inhibitors with or without *Helicobacter pylori* eradication if necessary.

2 E – Gastric adenocarcinoma

The incidence of gastric cancer reaches its peak between the ages of 50 and 70 years. Men are affected two to three times more than women. Epigastric pain with no specific relation to eating (and not relieved by antacids), early satiety/anorexia and dramatic weight loss are all symptoms associated with the disease. Depending on the site of the tumour other symptoms may include dysphagia (carcinoma at the cardia leading to oesophagogastric obstruction) or regurgitation of undigested food (cancer at the pylorus mimicking pyloric stenosis). A low haemoglobin and mean corpuscular volume attest to iron deficiency anaemia secondary to chronic blood loss.

3 J – Oesophageal varices

Oesophageal varices result from portal venous hypertension. This is most commonly the result of cirrhosis of the liver, usually associated with chronic alcohol abuse (note raised mean corpuscular volume because of the impact of alcohol on the bone marrow, and raised INR secondary to hepatic dysfunction, in this scenario). Porto-systemic shunting occurs as resistance to flow occurs and pressure rises in the portal venous system. In the significant, acute bleed clearly resuscitation must be implemented first – large-bore cannulae (central venous pressure line if possible), crystalloid or colloid immediately, with blood transfusion as soon as this is available. Fresh frozen plasma, vitamin K and platelets can be given if a coagulopathy is established, or if a large volume of blood needs to be replaced. Vasopressin/Terlipressin intravenously can help to markedly reduce portal venous pressure and slow or halt bleeding to allow a skilled endoscopist to band or inject the varices. If the bleeding remains torrential then tamponade using a Sengstaken–Blakemore tube can be attempted while definitive therapy or transfer are considered. Mortality from varices is high, not only because of the bleeding but as a result of the other disastrous complications of liver failure in alcoholics.

65 INVESTIGATION AND MANAGEMENT OF GASTROINTESTINAL PERFORATION

1 C – Conservative treatment (antibiotics, total parenteral nutrition, nasogastric tube)

There remains significant contention about operative versus non-operative management for oesophageal perforation. This is principally because surgical intervention implies the need for thoracotomy, a major plus procedure with high morbidity and lengthy recovery. There is general agreement that in the conservative management of instrumental oesophageal perforations, selection criteria should include small, localised leaks, with ready drainage back into the oesophagus (following contrast radiography), no pleural contamination and low-grade symptoms, with an absence of systemic signs of sepsis. As this man has presented late (> 3 days), he has theoretically undergone a selection process of sorts (ie if his perforation was more severe he would have deteriorated more rapidly). Conservative management includes the aggressive use of broad-spectrum antibiotics, parenteral nutrition and nasogastric suction with gastric acid suppression. Undoubtedly any clinical deterioration may cause revision of the plan for conservative therapy.

2 D – Computed tomography (CT) scan abdomen +/− guided drainage

This woman is demonstrating signs and symptoms of septically complicated diverticular disease (arising from micro- or macro-perforation). The management depends on the clinical scenario – simple diverticulitis does not usually require urgent radiological assessment and can be managed with bowel rest and antibiotics. The more ill patient, as in this case, should undergo contrast CT scanning to exclude free perforation and facilitate drainage of any abscess. The patient with generalised peritonitis in general requires a laparotomy.

66 JAUNDICE

1 I – Pancreatic carcinoma

The patient has presented with progressive symptoms suggestive of underlying pancreatic carcinoma. The finding of a palpable gallbladder may imply gallbladder pathology (eg gallstones). However, if Courvoisier's law ('if in the presence of jaundice the gallbladder is palpable, the cause is unlikely to be related to stones') is applied, the correct diagnosis is reached. The principle is that if the obstruction of the common bile duct is a stone, the gallbladder is usually fibrotic and therefore does not distend. Cholangiocarcinoma and multiple liver metastases can present similarly but the former is much less common than pancreatic cancer (this is therefore the more likely diagnosis) and the latter is associated with a palpable liver not gallbladder. Other characteristic symptoms of pancreatic cancer include severe abdominal and back pain. Investigations include ultrasound, computed tomography and endoscopic retrograde cholangiopancreatography and cytology.

2 F – Hepatocellular carcinoma

This accounts for approximately 90% of primary liver cancers, the typical presentation of which is illustrated in the case described. Associations include chronic infection with hepatitis B, cirrhosis and aflotoxin (*Aspergillus flavum*). Hepatocellular carcinoma may give rise to a solitary large mass or, rarely, multifocal nodules. The finding of a raised serum α-protein is highly suggestive, with diagnostic confirmation via percutaneous biopsy and histology.

3 J – Primary biliary cirrhosis

The presentation described is fairly typical for this disorder, 90% of cases are female and the peak age is 45–50 years. This autoimmune disorder is suspected from the typical pattern of the liver function tests, is confirmed by the finding of anti-mitochondrial antibodies/smooth muscle antibodies, and is proven by characteristic histology from liver biopsy. Associated disorders include thyroid disease and CREST (calcinosis, Raynaud phenomenon, oesophageal motility disorders, sclerodactyly, telangiectasia) syndrome. Treatment is symptomatic, eg nutritional support for malabsorption. Liver transplantation may be required.

67 DISORDERS OF THE PANCREAS

1 A – Acute pancreatitis

The patient's symptoms and signs are consistent with the diagnosis of acute pancreatitis. Of importance is the fact that a normal serum amylase concentration is not sufficiently sensitive to rule out the diagnosis. As in the case illustrated, late presentation makes this more likely; serum amylase typically peaks in the first 12–48 h and may return to normal after 72 h. In such cases the urinary amylase and serum lipase concentrations may be of value. Hypocalcaemia may occur in this potentially life-threatening disorder. The absence of previous episodes of pain, diabetes and symptoms suggestive of malabsorption make chronic pancreatitis unlikely. The diagnosis is confirmed on ultrasound and computed tomography scan findings.

2 H – Vipoma

These tumours are of APUD cells of the gastroenteropancreatic endocrine system. Patients tend to be middle-aged, with more women affected than men. Episodes of profuse watery diarrhoea are typical and continue even in the presence of fasting. Hypokalaemia occurs following excessive gastrointestinal secretion and symptoms of such may be the presenting feature. Vasoactive intestinal peptide (VIP) normally inhibits acid secretion; therefore, patients are hypochlorhydric or achlorhydric. Other abnormalities include hypercalcaemia and hyperglycaemia. Plasma VIP levels are elevated. Initial treatment is directed toward correcting volume and electrolyte abnormalities. Octreotide controls diarrhoea in 80% of cases. Both computed tomography and magnetic resonance imaging are of value in diagnosis and staging. Surgical exploration with tumour resection leads to cure in 50% of patients.

3 C – β-cell tumour of the pancreas

β-Cell tumour, or insulinoma, is the commonest form of islet cell tumour. Symptoms are related to hypoglycaemia and occur with increasing frequency and severity. Attacks may be more frequent in the early hours of the morning, with vague abdominal pain relieved by carbohydrates, hence the confusion with peptic ulcer disease. Episodes may similarly occur following exercise. The diagnosis is suggested by Whipple's triad, ie:

- attacks occurring in the fasting state
- during the height of the attack there is hypoglycaemia below 2.5 mmol/litre
- symptoms relieved by glucose.

Confirmation is by the identification of fasting hypoglycaemia associated with elevated levels of human insulin. Pancreatic angiography may aid in preoperative localisation with treatment by surgical excision of the tumour.

68 SCORING IN ACUTE PANCREATITIS

The commonest causes of acute pancreatitis are gallstones (50–60% of attacks in the UK) and alcohol. The rationale of a scoring system is to attempt to predict the presence of severe disease, to allow patient series to be compared, and to permit rational selection of patients for potential new treatment strategies. Ranson's score (HC Ranson, 1974) is commonly used and found in most textbooks (this is a multiple-factor scoring system based on a North American population with alcohol as the predominant aetiological factor). The Glasgow score is a modification of Ranson's scoring system, and was designed for use in a typical UK population with gallstone-predominant disease. Both of these systems are limited in that they cannot be completed immediately on admission; requiring 48 h of assessment. (A score of greater than 3 indicates severe disease.) The Acute Physiology and Chronic Health Evaluation (APACHE II, or more recently APACHE III) has the advantage of being able to be employed daily, but is extensive and time consuming (NB a score of > 8 implies severe disease). Biochemical scoring methods eg C-reactive protein and the Hong Kong system (based on glucose and urea); immunological scoring (interleukin-6); and radiological scoring (Balthazar–Ranson and computed tomography severity system) also exist.

1 I – Ranson score = 3

This scenario demonstrates the use of the Ranson scoring system. It looks at five specific criteria on admission and a further six criteria at 48 h. Mortality can be predicted on the result (0–2 < 5% mortality, 3–4 ~ 15–20%, 5–6 ~ 40%, > 6 ~ 100%). The three positive factors in this clinical case are white cell count > 16 on admission, haematocrit drop > 10% since admission and base excess < 4 at 48 h.

2 D – Glasgow score = 2

This presentation uses the Glasgow score to demonstrate disease severity. This is a nine-point scoring system. No haematocrit has been measured and no base deficit included. All tests were performed at the same time. Age > 55 and aspartate aminotransferase > 100 are the two positive criteria.

3 B – Balthazar–Ranson grading system

The distinction between interstitial and necrotising pancreatitis cannot be made unless intravenous contrast is used. A non-enhanced computed tomography (CT) does provide important information in accordance with the Balthazar–Ranson criteria of severity (graded A–E). When intravenous contrast is used a 'CT severity index' can be used. This index awards points on the basis of the CT grade and the amount of necrosis. (NB Patients with a combined score of 7–10 have a higher morbidity than those with a score < 7.)

69 COMPLICATIONS OF GALLSTONE DISEASE

When considering this subject, the candidate is advised to think of complications within and without the gallbladder, starting with the former and progressing to the ileum.

1 H – Gallstone ileus

This patient has symptoms typical of small bowel obstruction. Small bowel obstruction from impaction of a gallstone in the distal ileum is rare but most commonly occurs in women over 70 years old. It accounts for 20% of older patients with small bowel obstruction who do not have a history of a hernia or previous abdominal surgery. Plain abdominal films may show a classic triad of small bowel obstruction, a gallstone in the gut and gas in the biliary tree (although the Editor has yet to observe this in practice). Treatment is surgical with proximal enterotomy, removal of the stone, a search for further stones but not cholecystectomy (which is dangerous and unnecessary). A bonus mark could be given for this question for also choosing Mirizzi's syndrome because most patients also have a fistula.

2 B – Acute pancreatitis

The differential diagnosis is gallbladder perforation but this is much less common than pancreatitis. Typically patients present with severe upper abdominal pain radiating to the back, often associated with nausea and vomiting. Signs of cardiovascular or respiratory dysfunction may be present, abdominal signs range from mild epigastric or left upper quadrant tenderness to generalised peritonitis.

70 THE MANAGEMENT OF GALLSTONE DISEASE

The management of symptomatic gallstone disease has changed greatly over the last 20 years. It is an area of contention in many respects, and many algorithms exist (especially for the suspected bile duct stone) all of which have their merits. The final decision probably rests with the experience of the surgeon and the equipment available. The MRCS candidate might be advised to select the simplest and safest answer where doubt exists. These are given below.

1 A – ERCP and sphincterotomy

This lady is suffering from cholangitis as defined by Charcot's triad. The common bile duct is dilated (> 6–7 mm). She requires urgent drainage. This should be performed using ERCP with a laparoscopic cholecystectomy deferred to a later date. Failure to clear the duct by simple measures should prompt the use of a stent or, if this fails, transhepatic drainage (percutaneous transhepatic cholangiogram). Open surgical drainage is rarely required.

2 B – Early laparoscopic cholecystectomy +/− pre-operative cholangiography

This lady has acute cholecystitis with no evidence of common bile duct stones. The main choice lies between early (on the index admission) or interval cholecystectomy +/− pre-operative cholangiography. Opinion is divided but, increasingly, surgery is being advocated on the index admission. This is in the acceptance that although the rate of conversion to open surgery is high (20% approximately), it is similarly high at a later date and further complications, including further episodes of inflammation, occur with regularity while on the waiting list.

3 I – Percutaneous (radiological) gallbladder drainage

In a fit person, empyema of the gallbladder (as presented here) might be managed by emergency open cholecystectomy. Before the advent of interventional radiology, if experience was not available, laparotomy could be performed with open drainage. The best treatment, however, in this case would be radiological drainage with antibiotics/resuscitative measures, which will hopefully rectify the situation without recourse to life-threatening surgery.

71 RECTAL BLEEDING

1 I – Infective colitis

Cytomegalovirus colitis can cause severe diarrhoea and torrential, even life-threatening, rectal bleeding. This diagnosis should always be considered first in patients on immunosuppression. This and other infections are common problems in acquired immune deficiency syndrome – other responsible organisms include herpes virus, and *Cryptosporidium.*

2 H – Haemorrhoids

Bright-red rectal bleeding in a young patient is invariably the result of haemorrhoids. Such bleeding is often triggered by trauma leading to ulceration of previously asymptomatic small piles. This can often be confirmed on proctoscopy in the acute phase but quite often you see the patient in outpatients weeks or months later when the problem has completely resolved. No further action need be taken.

3 C – Angiodysplasia

These are a type of arteriovenous malformation and are one of the common causes of significant lower gastrointestinal bleeding in the elderly population. As in this case, it is notoriously difficult to pinpoint the actual offending vessel. Where direct vision fails, mesenteric angiography or radionucleotide scans can sometimes be of diagnostic use but often also yield negative results if the vessel is not actively bleeding at the time of investigation. Should angiography demonstrate the source of bleeding, therapeutic embolisation can be performed. In cases of continued bleeding with negative investigations, treatment may involve total colectomy as a life-saving measure.

72 CONSTIPATION

Constipation is the second most common gastrointestinal symptom in the developed world. In most patients, low fluid intake, low dietary fibre, and lack of exercise or mobility may contribute to 'simple' constipation. However, constipation may be caused by 'organic' pathology when it occurs secondary to structural or systemic abnormalities. Organic causes may affect the gastrointestinal tract itself, eg mechanical obstruction secondary to carcinoma/stricture, and persistent dilatation of the bowel (megabowel) occurring without obvious cause (idiopathic) or secondary to Hirschsprung disease. Extragastrointestinal pathology may also cause constipation. Examples include endocrine/metabolic, neurological and psychological disorders. Constipation may also occur secondary to certain medication (opiates, antidepressants, anticholinergics, anticonvulsants). In the absence of an organic cause for constipation, the term 'functional' constipation is adopted to indicate disordered function of the hindgut. On the basis of physiological investigations, such patients may be divided into those with a delay in transit through all or part of the colon (slow transit constipation), and/or those with abnormalities of rectal evacuation (outlet obstruction) or those with no abnormality (constipation-predominant irritable bowel syndrome). The causes in the list provided may be classified using this system to provide a comprehensive differential diagnosis for constipation.

1 N – Outlet obstruction

This patient has 'functional constipation', because investigations have excluded an organic cause. Constipation may refer to the infrequent and/or difficult passage of stools. A predominance of symptoms of difficult evacuation, which is often referred to as obstructed defaecation (eg excessive straining, a sensation of incomplete evacuation, digitation etc) is suggestive of outlet obstruction, rather than slow transit constipation, although physiological confirmation is required as symptoms do *not* accurately predict underlying pathophysiology. The history of perineal massage and a 'bulge' in the vagina (posterior wall) is suggestive of the presence of a rectocoele, which may lead to outlet obstruction, as a result of redistribution of evacuatory forces during defaecation.

2 A – Colorectal carcinoma

This diagnosis must always be excluded in patients presenting with altered bowel habit. It is now clear that most patients with colorectal cancer who present with altered bowel habit report loose stools or diarrhoea. This represents 'overflow' of proximal bowel content because of narrowing of the lumen in the affected segment of bowel. Careful history taking often reveals a period of constipation preceding the change in stool consistency. It is unwise to attribute potentially sinister symptoms (eg bleeding per rectum) to 'benign' pathology (eg haemorrhoids) until proximal pathology has been excluded.

3 J – Idiopathic megabowel

Persistent dilatation of the bowel is known as megabowel. This may occur secondary to an absence of ganglion cells in the myenteric plexus (Hirschsprung disease), where failure of relaxation of the affected segment leads to gross proximal dilatation. Alternatively, no obvious cause may be identifiable, when it is termed idiopathic megabowel. This condition is characterised by severe infrequency of defaecation, with several weeks between bowel movements. There is usually associated passive leakage of stool as a result of 'overflow' around impacted stool in the rectum. The diagnosis is confirmed on barium enema, which reveals dilatation of the rectum, and sometimes colon. Management involves behavioural, medical and, rarely, surgical treatment.

73 DIARRHOEA

1 N – Ulcerative colitis

Interestingly, both ulcerative colitis and irritable bowel syndrome (IBS) appear to be triggered in a proportion of patients following acute enteritis (the entity of post-infectious IBS is well established). The symptoms and signs are those of an acute attack of colitis confirmed by sigmoidoscopy. Clearly, before steroids are administered, stool culture must be performed, however, as in this case.

2 D – Crohn's disease

This patient (on balance) has evidence of Crohn's colitis. This is supported by rectal sparing and skip lesions within the colon. It is not infrequent for biopsies to have insufficient findings to conclusively support a diagnosis either of Crohn's disease or ulcerative colitis and these are usually described as indeterminate.

74 TYPES OF COLITIS

1 A – Collagenous colitis

This is an uncommon form of colitis and is part of the disease spectrum termed microscopic colitis (the other main subdivision is lymphocytic). It is most common among middle-aged women and there is an association with autoimmune disorders such as coeliac disease, thyroid disorders, diabetes and rheumatoid arthritis. Patients typically present with symptoms and signs of colitis, as in the case described. Stool and blood investigations tend to be normal. Endoscopic examination of the bowel similarly appears normal to the naked eye and the disorder is generally diagnosed on histological examination of biopsies taken at endoscopy – hence the name, microscopic colitis. No cure is yet available. Treatment is directed at reducing inflammation and the symptoms of diarrhoea by means of drugs such as sulphasalazine and mesalazine. Short courses of steroids may be required for severe cases.

2 E – Ischaemic colitis

The case describes the classical triad of acute onset of abdominal pain, rectal bleeding and shock in an elderly patient. The patient may have atrial fibrillation or another factor such as cardiac or liver disease. Treatment involves resuscitation with intravenous fluids, blood and blood products before laparotomy, at which the affected segment of bowel is resected. However, this may not be possible if the whole of the mesenteric supply is affected (superior mesenteric occlusion with infarction of the small bowel and right side of the colon).

3 I – Ulcerative colitis

DALMs (dysplasia-associated lesion or mass) are polyps with surrounding dysplasia that can occur in chronic ulcerative colitis. They are significant indicators of carcinoma elsewhere in the bowel or at least its imminent development. They are therefore a strong indication for colectomy.

75 INVESTIGATION OF DISORDERS OF THE LARGE INTESTINE

1 D – Colonoscopy

When assessing a patient's risk of developing colorectal cancer (CRC), the family history is of paramount importance. A family history of CRC in a first-degree relative is a significant finding and the age at which the diagnosis was made is similarly of importance when quantifying a patient's overall relative risk. So an individual with a first-degree relative diagnosed with CRC earlier than age 55 years has a relative risk that is two- to five-fold above that of individuals without a family history of CRC. In this case, the patient is categorised as at moderate risk of developing CRC during her lifetime and as such this warrants screening by colonoscopy. Moderate risk is defined as having:

- one first-degree relative affected by CRC before the age of 45 years
- two (one aged less than 55 years) or three relatives at any age affected by CRC or endometrial carcinoma who are first-degree relatives of each other and one a first-degree relative of the patient
- two affected first-degree relatives (one aged less than 55 years).

2 D – Colonoscopy

Complete examination of the colon is warranted as this patient is at a high risk of having synchronous adenomatous polyps and/or colorectal carcinoma. This is on the basis of the findings of an adenomatous polyp > 1 cm in diameter and villous histology. Other criteria include multiple (more than two) adenomas and adenomas with high-grade dysplasia. The incidence of a synchronous lesion in such a case is of the order of 2%. Such lesions may be detected by barium enema examination; however, colonoscopy has the advantage of allowing endoscopic polypectomy to be performed. So it is not only diagnostic, but also therapeutic. Further follow-up colonoscopy timings are outlined in the British Society of Gastroenterology (BSG) guidelines and depend on the findings.

3 J – Mesenteric angiography

Mesenteric angiography is the logical next step in the management of a patient in whom colonoscopy has failed to detect the source of bleeding. This is of particular importance in an elderly patient who has evidence of significant ongoing bleeding, but who is cardiovascularly stable. Angiography relies on active bleeding for diagnosis, following which therapeutic embolisation of the offending vessel may be performed. Should the investigation fail to demonstrate the cause, and the patient continue to bleed, then laparotomy and colectomy may be nescassary as a life-saving procedure.

4 E – Computed tomography (CT) scan of chest, abdomen and pelvis

This patient has beeen diagnosed with colorectal carcinoma and as such the next step is to stage the disease process. This requires imaging of the liver and chest for metastatic disease. Isolated ultrasound scanning of the liver is insufficient and in fact the use of CT is recommended in national cancer services guidelines. Were the tumour to be rectal, magnetic resonance imaging of the pelvis should also be performed for local 'T' staging.

5 M – Water-soluble contrast enema

Although the vignette strongly points to malignant large bowel obstruction, and a laparotomy will almost certainly, therefore, be required, it is imperative to exclude pseudo-obstruction before risking a potentially unnecessary laparotomy. This can be achieved by an enema or by computed tomography scan with rectal contrast. In modern practice, it may also identify whether a stent can be deployed, especially in unfit elderly patients.

76 FAECAL INCONTINENCE

The aetiology of faecal incontinence should be thought of as a disturbance to the passage or passenger. The 'passage' consists of the rectum, which stores and expels faeces when appropriate, and the anal canal which is composed of two rings of muscle (the internal and external anal sphincter) that relax to allow emptying. The pudenal nerve is a mixed nerve that provides motor function to the external anal sphincter, as well as sensation to the anal canal providing sensory input that forms part of a 'sampling reflex'. The 'passenger' or faeces, if loose, will frequently result in incontinence even in the presence of a normally functioning anorectal sphincteric complex (as anyone who has experienced severe dysentery would know). Alternatively, sphincteric disruption may lead to incontinence even for normal stool.

1 G – Sphincter disruption

Obstetric trauma frequently results in a transient degree of faecal incontinence in the immediate post-partum period in up to a third of women but this incontinence subsequently improves. This is related to traction of the sphincteric complex and the pudendal nerve. An alarming proportion of women sustain occult sphincteric damage and evidence suggests that many third-degree tears (extending from perineum to involve the anal sphincter complex) are inadequately repaired.

2 A – Colorectal carcinoma

In this case the 'passenger' is responsible for causing faecal incontinence. This scenario highlights the importance of excluding all organic pathology in a patient who has few other symptoms indicating that they have a carcinoma. Any new symptoms or change in bowel habit in a patient over 45 years old should prompt thorough examination and investigation, before assessing for a functional pathology.

3 F – Pudendal neuropathy

Multiple, traumatic vaginal deliveries will result in a stretch injury to the pudendal nerve. This results in a weakness in the external anal sphincter, causing attenuated squeeze pressure. Patients subsequently complain of an inability to defer defaecation (urgency) with incontinence. This lady might benefit from a low-dose of amitryptiline, which has been demonstrated to reduce rectal sensitivity, and biofeedback. In the absence of a discrete sphincteric lesion, there are few surgical procedures that have sustained benefit. In extreme cases, a colostomy may be the only option available to such patients.

77 FISTULA-IN-ANO (CLASSIFICATION)

Successful surgical management of anal fistulae depends upon accurate knowledge of anal sphincter anatomy and the fistula's course through it. Failure to understand either may result in fistula recurrence or incontinence. The most comprehensive and practical classification is that devised by St Mark's Hospital. Sir Alan Parks's cryptoglandular hypothesis (1976) is central, holding first that the majority of fistulae arise from an abscess in the intersphincteric plane, and second that the relation of the primary tract to the external sphincter is paramount in surgical management. The classic diagram of various fistulae is a favourite of vivas where you might be asked to reproduce it.

1 E – Mid-transsphincteric

Transsphincteric fistulae have a primary tract that passes through both sphincters at varying levels into the ischiorectal fossa where they may lead to ischiorectal abscess formation. The fistula may be described as high, mid- or low depending on where the fistula crosses the external sphincter, ie above, at, or below the level of the dentate line respectively.

2 C – Intersphincteric

Sepsis having developed within the intersphincteric plane, it follows the path of least resistance down the intersphincteric space, emerging at the peri-anal skin, resulting in an intersphincteric fistula (and often presenting acutely as a peri-anal abscess).

3 A – Extrasphincteric

These rare fistulae run without relation to the sphincters and are classified according to their pathology. They often originate from a segment of sigmoid diverticular disease or from ileal or sigmoid Crohn's disease. They can also be created by injudicious probing of peri-anal sepsis (iatrogenic).

78 TREATMENT OF BENIGN ANORECTAL DISORDERS

1 E – Fistulotomy

This patient has an intersphincteric anal fistula. Successful surgical management of anal fistulae depends upon accurate knowledge of anal sphincter anatomy and the fistula's course through it; failure to understand either may result in fistula recurrence or incontinence. This patient's fistula is amenable to fistulotomy (a procedure with a > 90% success rate), as it only encircles a proportion of the internal sphincter muscle fibres which when laid open are unlikely to result in significant continence disturbance.

2 C – Diltiazem ointment

This patient has an anal fissure the initial management of which is medical. 50–70% of patients who apply 0.2% glyceryl trinitrate ointment three times daily for 8 weeks have significant symptomatic improvement/healing. Unfortunately, one of the side-effects is severe headaches which may result in poor patient compliance. In this situation 2% diltiazem ointment, which is equally efficacious but more expensive, is recommended.

3 H – Haemorrhoidectomy

Small internal (bleeding) or prolapsing haemorrhoids above the dentate line can be treated by injection sclerotherapy or rubber-band ligation, respectively. Haemorrhoids refractory to non-operative therapy, or those that are large and prolapsing with a significant external component usually require haemorrhoidectomy. There are essentially two commonly used surgical options: Milligan and Morgan's sharp (now usually diathermy) excision and stapled haemorrhoidectomy (PPH). The patient should of course be appraised of the risks before embarking on surgery.

79 DISEASES OF THE ANUS

1 C – Anal fissure

This is the typical presentation of this condition.

2 A, B, or E

Infection with human papillomavirus can lead to anal warts (molluscum contagiosum) and dysplastic changes within the anal epithelium (mild to severe: termed anal epithelial neoplasia). These may progress to anal carcinoma. So patients with warts and those with other sexually transmitted diseases affecting the anus should have biopsies and possibly thence surveillance if required.

3 K – Proctalgia fugax

This is defined as episodic, intense anal pain of short duration (usually at night) in which all other disorders have been excluded. Proctalgia fugax occurs in up to 18% of the US population, being more common in men, and those < 40 years old. It is thought to be secondary to sensory dysfunction, with possible hypersensitivity of the internal anal sphincter and rectal musculature, precipitated by psychological stress. Treatment can be problematic with many systemic (eg antidepressants) and local (eg glyceryl trinitrate) remedies tried.

Breast/endocrine surgery

80 BREAST LUMPS

1 A – Breast abscess

This is the classical history of the presentation of a breast abscess. More commonly seen in the lactating mother (infective organisms can penetrate the breast through a crack in the nipple) they are usually caused by infection with *Staphylococcus aureus.* Once an abscess has formed there is no place for antibiotic treatment alone as this will simply result in the formation of an 'antibioma' (a chronic, sterile abscess). Instead initial treatment should be via daily ultrasound-guided aspiration of the abscess with concomitant antimicrobial therapy. If this fails then formal surgical drainage will be necessary.

2 C – Fibroadenoma

This young woman has clinical, histological and radiological signs of a fibroadenoma (sometimes called a 'breast mouse' on account of its mobility). Fibroadenoma is a benign breast disorder and is a developmental aberration of lobular development. Any organ in the body that undergoes cyclical changes of proliferation and regression can be subject to disorders of these processes. To appropriately reflect this the nomenclature of benign breast disease refers to the processes as 'aberrations of normal development and involution' or ANDI (described by the Cardiff Breast Clinic). The umbrella of ANDI covers cyclical mastalgia and nodularity, cyst formation, sclerosing adenosis, duct ectasia, fibroadenoma and papilloma formation. Surgical excision should be offered in women over 35, or if the lump is over 4 cm in size. In the under 35s excision or reassessment should be proffered dependent on patient wishes (anxiety etc). Cancer risk in a fibroadenoma is 1/1000 (usually lobular carcinoma *in situ*).

3 B – Breast cyst

Cysts usually present as discrete, painful swellings, often with sudden onset. Cysts fall into the category of ANDI (see above) as they represent aberrations of lobular involution. They are commonly seen in peri-menopausal women, and can be multiple and involve both breasts. Fine-needle aspiration of a cyst reveals fluid that can be green, yellow, or brown in colour. If the fluid is blood-stained and, after aspiration, a mass remains at the site of the swelling, malignancy must be suspected. In such cases the fluid should be sent for cytology and a mammogram should be performed.

4 F – Invasive ductal carcinoma

The clinical presentation clearly points to a diagnosis of breast cancer. The cytological grading, C5 (malignant cells) confirms this. The features of this lump that make it more likely to be a ductal carcinoma rather than a lobular one are:

- presence of a single lesion (multiple and bilateral lesions are more likely in lobular cancer)
- branching microcalcification visible on mammography
- increased incidence of ductal carcinoma versus lobular (75–80% of cases versus 10–15% of cases respectively).

81 MASTALGIA

1 A – Acute mastitis

The commonest form of mastitis is that occuring in relation to pregnancy and breastfeeding, the so called 'lactational mastitis'. The condition is more common among smokers. Most cases are caused by *Staphylococcus aureus* when an ascending infection from the nipple, along the lactiferous ducts, initiates the mastitis. In the early phase the spreading cellulitis produces the classical signs of inflammation. After a few days an abscess develops, which may give rise to a palpable lump. The time-scale and the absence of a lump, either clinically or radiologically, differentiates acute mastitis from a breast abscess. Treatment is with antibiotics alone.

2 I – Tietze's syndrome

Tietze's syndrome is an inflammatory condition of the costochondral cartilages. It is characterised by pain, tenderness and swelling of one or more costal cartilages, typically the first four. The syndrome usually affects older children and young adults and there are more female cases than male cases. The pain is usually exacerbated by physical activity, deep inspiration and coughing. Examination reveals the presence of exquisite tenderness and swelling over the affected joints. Treatment consists of local heat, analgesics, anti-inflammatory drugs, or local steroid injections. Most often the pain subsides after a few weeks or months but swelling may persist for longer.

3 D – Breast carcinoma

Pain is an uncommon feature of breast carcinoma; however, when it does occur it is typically described as an ache or prickling sensation in the breast. This tends to draw the patient's attention to the more common complaint of a lump in the breast.

82 NIPPLE DISCHARGE

Up to two-thirds of all normal non-lactating women produce fluid from the nipple if a small amount of negative-pressure is applied, and this varies from yellow to dark green. However, it is never blood-stained. Management is influenced by triple assessment, comprising clinical assessment, imaging and cytology. Haemo-Stix is an easy bedside test used to test for the presence of blood in discharge.

1 E – Mammary duct ectasia

Duct ectasia or duct dilatation can occur as part of the normal involution process of the breast. Symptomatic duct ectasia is benign and should therefore be considered as an aberration of this normal process. In the past, peri-ductal mastitis was thought to be the same disease process, but this has since been demonstrated as a separate pathological entity. Duct ectasia usually affects women between the ages of 50 and 60 years, and patients present as described in the scenario with nipple retraction and discharge. It is rarely frankly blood-stained and is often multiductal. The majority of patients have normal mammograms, although some radiographs can demonstrate duct thickening and coarse retro-alveolar calcification.

2 G – Mammary intraductal papilloma

The lesion is benign but associated with an increased risk of developing an invasive breast carcinoma. Patients present clinically either with serous or bloody nipple discharge, or with a small sub-areolar tumour. Mammography may be abnormal as described although there may also be no lesion seen. Treatment involves microdochectomy, usually performed following the insertion of a fine probe into the affected duct while the patient is awake. A total duct excision may be performed if there are multiple ducts involved, but this is associated with a 20% risk of loss of nipple sensation.

3 H – Peri-ductal mastitis

This question highlights that men also suffer from benign breast disease. As mentioned earlier, peri-ductal mastitis has, in the past, been mistakenly confused with duct ectasia. Peri-ductal mastitis is characterised by peri-areolar inflammation, a non-lactating breast abscess, or a mammary duct fistula. Patients may also describe severe breast pain. An important distinguishing aetiological factor in peri-ductal mastitis is smoking; 90% of affected women are smokers compared with 38% in an unaffected age-matched population. Treatment involves drainage of any underlying abscess, antibiotic treatment and, in recurrent cases, excision of the affected tissue. Care needs to be taken because drainage may result in fistula formation, and co-incidental malignancy needs to be excluded.

4 B – Epithelial hyperplasia

Epithelial hyperplasia is described as an increase in the number of layers of lining epithelial cells in the terminal duct lobular unit. If there is evidence of atypia in the cells, then this is known as atypical hyperplasia, and is associated with a four to five times increased risk of breast cancer compared with the normal population. However, some mild epithelial hyperplasia is a normal variant seen in pre-menopausal breast tissue. Atypical hyperplasia is further divided into atypical lobular or ductal hyperplasia, dependent on histological findings and not on origins of the cells. Women with atypical ductal hyperplasia who have a first-degree relative with breast cancer have a 20–30% absolute risk of developing breast cancer over the following 20 years. Patients with atypical lobular hyperplasia are likely to develop cancer with an equal frequency in either breast, compared to patients with ductal hyperplasia, which tends to be confined to the breast in which it is biopsied. Although the answer to this scenario may have been breast carcinoma, this rarely presents with simply nipple discharge.

83 GYNAECOMASTIA

Gynaecomastia may be physiological when it is seen in newborn infants, pubescent adolescents and elderly individuals. Pathological gynaecomastia may result from decreased production and/or action of testosterone, increased production and/or action of oestrogen, or drug use. It may also be idiopathic in nature. Decreased production of testosterone may be the result of primary or secondary hypogonadism (gonadotrophin deficiency, eg pituitary disorders). Increased production and/or action of oestrogen can occur at the testicular level or at the periphery as a result of production by testicular tumours or of ectopic production of human chorionic gonadotrophin (eg by carcinoma of lung, kidney, gastrointestinal tract and by extragonadal germ cell tumours). In addition, it may arise as a result of peripheral conversion, which can be because of increased substrate or increased activity of aromatase as in chronic liver disease, malnutrition, hyperthyroidism, adrenal tumours and familial gynaecomastia. Oestrogen-secreting tumours of the adrenal gland are an exceptionally rare cause of gynaecomastia.

1 D – Genetic

This patient has Kallman's syndrome, which is characterised by hypothalamic gonadotrophin-releasing hormone (GnRH) deficiency and deficient olfactory sense – hyposmia or anosmia. It is usually inherited as an X-linked or autosomal recessive disorder, although new mutations may arise. Gonadotrophin deficiency arises from a failure of embryonic migration of GnRH-secreting neurones from their site of origin in the nose. The same defect affects the olfactory neurones, resulting in olfactory bulb aplasia. More than half of patients have associated somatic stigmata, most commonly, nerve deafness, colour blindness, mid-line cranio-facial deformities such as cleft lip and palate, and renal abnormalities. Anosmia can be demonstrated using simple stimuli such as cloves, peppermint and eucalyptus. Serum luteinising hormone and follicle-stimulating hormone levels are low. Klinefelter's syndrome (XXY) is another genetic cause.

2 F – Iatrogenic drug therapy

The clinical scenario describes a patient with onset of gynaecomastia following medical treatment of prostate cancer, which employs the use of anti-androgen drugs such as cyproterone acetate or flutamide. Various drugs are implicated in gynecomastia and can be classified into the following categories:

- oestrogens or drugs with oestrogen-like activity, such as diethylstilboestrol, digitalis and oestrogen-contaminated food and oestrogen-containing cosmetics
- drugs that enhance oestrogen synthesis, such as gonadotrophins, clomiphene and phenytoin
- drugs that inhibit testosterone synthesis or action, such as ketoconazole, metronidazole, alkylating agents, cisplatin, spironolactone, cimetidine, flutamide, finasteride and etomidate.

3 C – Chronic renal failure

The diagnosis is evident because of the long-history of type I diabetes. The presence of scars on the forearms (arteriovenous fistula formation for haemodialysis) and the sub-umbilical region (insertion of catheters for peritoneal dialysis) confirm that the patient has end-stage renal failure requiring dialysis. Such patients may develop gynaecomastia, and this is thought to be the result of a combination of increased luteinising hormone and oestrogen levels.

84 MANAGEMENT OF BREAST CANCER

1 I – Wide local excision and axillary clearance

Breast conservation surgery is considered the optimal therapy for local treatment of breast cancer and commonly takes the form of a wide local excision for local treatment of breast cancer. When combined with post-operative radiotherapy the results are comparable to mastectomy. Indications for wide local excision include:

- stage I or II disease
- single primary lesion
- tumours < 4 cm in diameter (this is because poor cosmetic results often follow wide local excision for tumours > 4cm; however tumours over 4 cm may be treated by wide local excision if the breast is large).

Evidence of vascular invasion requires not only local treatment, but also treatment directed towards the axillary lymph nodes. This is most commonly performed by means of an axillary clearance. Following surgery, the patient should be referred for consideration of chemotherapy. Note: the practice of sentinel node biopsy is becoming a popular alternative and is now in fact recommended in every woman with breast cancer (RCS guidelines). Using a dye technique, if the sentinel node is found to be cancer-free women can be spared axillary surgery.

2 C – Chemotherapy

Combination chemotherapy reduces the annual odds of recurrence and death. The absolute benefits are greatest for women with node-positive disease. Furthermore, chemotherapy should be discussed with and offered to woman with node-negative but grade III (poorly differentiated) tumours. It is uncertain as to which regimen is best and there are several ongoing trials. At present the commonest combination is cyclophosphamide, methotrexate and 5-fluorouracil (CMF).

3 J – Wire-guided wide local excision

Treatment of screen-detected lesions differs from palpable breast cancer in that radiological localisation by means of a wire inserted into the lesion is required before excision. This patient has ductal carcinoma *in situ* (DCIS), the majority of which are now detected in screening programmes. In patients with extensive DCIS (> 4 cm) or disease affecting more than one quadrant a mastectomy should be performed. Surgical staging of the axilla is not required. Following adequate local excision of DCIS, patients should be considered for radiotherapy to the breast, which may reduce the risk of recurrence and development of invasive breast cancer.

4 G – Tamoxifen

The situation described is not unusual and management of locally advanced (stage III) disease involves treatment with systemic therapy. This may take the form of chemotherapy or hormonal treatment. Surgery and/or radiotherapy should normally be given afterwards, the timing of which is dependent on response to therapy. In patients who are unfit for surgery and who are unsuitable candidates for chemotherapy (as in the case described), the aim of therapy is to control the primary tumour while maintaining the best quality of life. In this instance, primary treatment is with tamoxifen provided the receptor status of the tumour is known. Anastrozole (Arimidex) is used as a second-line treatment.

5 F – Radiotherapy

Treatment with radiotherapy is mandatory in the case of a young woman who has undergone breast conservation surgery. This is usually started 2–4 weeks post-operatively, provided that wounds have healed and an adequate local excision has been performed (clear lateral margins of > 1 mm). The extent of the margin needs to be balanced against the final cosmetic appearance; however, any margin that is incomplete, ie < 1 mm, requires further excision before radiotherapy.

85 MISCELLANEOUS DISORDERS OF THE FEMALE BREAST

1 G – Mondor's disease

In a patient complaining of sudden breast pain, the finding of a tender subcutaneous cord, attached to the skin, is pathognomic of Mondor's disease. This rare condition is characterised by a sclerosing thrombophlebitis of the subcutaneous veins of the anterior chest wall, which give rise to the clinical findings. Imaging studies tend to be unremarkable. The condition is benign and self-limiting although a fibrous subcutaneous band may remain. Treatment is symptomatic with non-steroidal anti-inflammatories.

86 THYROID SWELLINGS

1 A – Anaplastic carcinoma

The acute presentation, in a woman of this age, with concomitant lymphadenopathy and a euthyroid profile, indicates a diagnosis of anaplastic carcinoma. This aggressive tumour accounts for 5–14% of primary thyroid neoplasms. Peak incidence is in the 7th decade (60–80 years); 30% arising in a long-standing goitre. Rapid local spread occurs, leading to compression and invasion of the trachea, and symptoms of upper oesophageal narrowing (eg dysphagia). There is usually early dissemination to the cervical lymph nodes (deep cervical nodes may be palpably enlarged) and vascular spread can occur to the lungs, skeleton and brain. By the time of presentation, unfortunately, most of these tumours are inoperable and the prognosis is dismal. Palliative radiotherapy and tracheostomy may be required for local symptom control.

2 L – Papillary carcinoma

The diagnosis in this case is that of papillary carcinoma. This is the commonest form of thyroid cancer, accounting for 60–80% of all thyroid neoplasms. These tumours are slow growing and arise predominantly in young adults, adolescents and even children. There is a 50% spread to local lymph nodes on presentation. Treatment is controversial. As disease can be multifocal and bilateral some feel that a total thyroidectomy should be undertaken; however, morbidity is clearly much more significant with this operation. Lobectomy with isthmusectomy is usually the procedure carried out in the lower risk groups, and prognosis is good when used in conjunction with suppressive doses of thyroxine (NB papillary tumours are thyroid-stimulating hormone-dependent and thyroxine reduces the risk of recurrence.)

3 F – Haemorrhage into a cyst

This history of prior neck swelling, acute pain and symptoms of tracheal compression; with a euthyroid biochemical profile, suggest that this young lady has had a haemorrhage into a thyroid cyst. Acute management involves ensuring airway patency and may be achieved by simple aspiration of the blood from the cyst. However, more extreme symptoms that fail to respond to aspiration will require emergency surgical intervention. Because of the risk of haemorrhage into a cyst, and also the small chance of toxic or malignant change in the gland, young patients are often advised to undergo thyroidectomy and subsequently take replacement hormone therapy.

87 DISEASES OF THE THYROID GLAND

1 C – De Quervain's thyroiditis

Inflammatory changes of the thyroid are common and may not be reflected in a change in the actual function of the gland. Thyroiditis can be divided into acute, subacute (de Quervain's), Hashimoto's thyroiditis (associated with hypothyroidism) and Reidel's thyroiditis. De Quervain's thyroiditis is primarily caused by a viral infection, such as mumps, Epstein–Barr or influenza, with a prodromal episode as described in the scenario. The gland may become enlarged up to three times its usual size but remains soft, distinguishing it from Reidel's (fibrosing) thyroiditis. In this latter condition a dense fibrosis results from the inflammation, which prompted Reidel in 1896 to describe this as 'inflammation of mysterious nature producing an iron-hard tumefaction of the thyroid'. In de Quervain's thyroiditis, 50% of patients demonstrate transient signs of mild hyperthyroidism as a result of the release of thyroxine from damaged thyroid parenchyma. However, thyroid function often returns to normal although a small percentage of patients subsequently become mildly hypothyroid as the gland shrinks. The hyperthyroidism can be differentiated from Graves' disease by the low uptake on scintiscanning. Usually no clinical treatment is required for de Quervain's thyroiditis, although non-steroidal anti-inflammatory drugs may ease initial discomfort.

2 L – Sick euthyroidism

This man is critically unwell and it is not uncommon for such patients to demonstrate a low T_3 and T_4 but normal TSH. This forms part of a stress reaction but in the presence of a normal TSH, this would not be classed as a true hypothyroidism.

88 COMPLICATIONS OF THYROIDECTOMY

1 E – Hypocalcaemia

Hypocalcaemia after thyroidectomy may occur for two reasons: metabolic and anatomical. Metabolic causes are not fully understood but may be secondary to the release of calcitonin during manipulation or a reduction of renal tubular resorption of calcium without a change in parathormone or calcitonin levels. Anatomical causes are the result of excision of all parathyroid tissue during total thyroidectomy. If the calcium is > 2.0 mmol/litre, symptoms usually resolve within 2 days without treatment. If symptoms persist or worsen treatment with calcium supplementation and synthetic vitamin D will be necessary.

2 N – Thyroid storm

This is a rare but life-threatening condition precipitated by thyroid surgery, infection, stress, or radioactive iodine therapy in an unprepared patient. It is caused by the sudden release of massive amounts of thyroid hormone into the systemic circulation resulting in hyperpyrexia, tachycardia, extreme restlessness, diarrhoea and vomiting. It may mimic the acute abdomen but needs emergency treatment. Assessment and appropriate management of the airways, breathing and circulation should be performed. Fluid resuscitation with normal saline is required with propanolol together with potassium iodide, carbimazole and dexamethasone.

3 G – Superior laryngeal nerve paralysis

Damage to the superior laryngeal nerve can cause voice weakness or fatigue, mild hoarseness and loss of vocal range. The upper half octave in range is lost, which can be particularly troublesome for singers, and is unlikely to be recovered.

4 D – Bilateral incomplete recurrent laryngeal nerve paralysis

Recurrent laryngeal nerve damage may be uni- or bilateral secondary to bruising, stretching, division devascularisation or ligation. In bilateral incomplete recurrent laryngeal nerve paralysis both vocal cords lie in the midline, unable to abduct, and there is severe dyspnoea with stridor soon after operation. Tracheal collapse (secondary to tracheomalacia) and haemorrhage into the pre-tracheal space may both present similarly; however, the former is rare and the latter usually evident on examination. In bilateral complete recurrent laryngeal nerve paralysis the two vocal cords occupy the cadaveric position, midway between the normal resting position and the midline. No abduction or adduction is possible; the voice is lost, but the dyspnoea is not severe. In unilateral complete recurrent laryngeal nerve paralysis all the laryngeal muscles on the affected side are paralysed except the cricothyroid and part of the arytenoideus. The affected cord lies in the cadaveric position; the opposite cord can be adducted, but the differences in vocal cord tension produce a hoarse voice. Unilateral incomplete recurrent laryngeal nerve paralysis produces slight dyspnoea on exertion and little or no alteration in the voice.

89 DISORDERS OF CALCIUM HOMEOSTASIS

When assessing calcium values it is important to establish albumin levels because only 40% of total calcium is ionised and therefore physiologically relevant. The remainder is bound to albumin and so unavailable to tissues. Routine laboratory values usually measure total plasma calcium and this must be corrected for the serum albumin concentration. This is done by adding or subtracting 0.02 mmol/litre for every g/litre by which the albumin lies below or above 40 g/litre. For critical values, the sample should be taken from an uncuffed arm with the patient in the fasting state to reduce variability in the protein values.

1 G – Hypoparathyroidism

This woman is truly hypocalcaemic, given her normal albumin levels, and needs urgent treatment. Her hypocalcaemia may be the result of removal of the dominant gland (so leaving under-active tissue) of oedema, damage to the remaining glands, or indeed of inadvertent surgical removal of all the parathyroid glands. She requires immediate intravenous 10 ml calcium gluconate given slowly over 5 min with cardiac monitoring. This infusion then needs to be repeated with 40 ml over 24 h. Maintenance therapy is achieved with 1α-(OH)D_3 or 1,25(OH)D_3. The most common general cause of hypocalcaemia, however, is renal failure. Signs include Chvostek's and Trousseau's: the former being twitching of the facial muscles induced by tapping over the facial nerve, and the latter being a carpopedal spasm caused by occluding the brachial artery.

2 F – Hyperparathyroidism

This woman demonstrates two of the symptoms of hypercalcaemia, which are renal calculi or calcification, bone pain, muscle weakness, intestinal atony, psychosis, peptic ulceration and pancreatitis ('stones, groans and psychic moans'). The list of causes of hypercalcaemia is extensive, however, in an otherwise well patient, the two most likely diagnoses are primary hyperparathyroidism or malignancy. The latter appears unlikely, and a diagnosis of hyperparathyroidism can be made on estimation of parathyroid hormone levels. Hyperparathyroidism is described as being primary, secondary, or tertiary. Primary is usually caused by a single parathyroid adenoma, rarely a carcinoma. Secondary is seen as a physiological response to hypocalcaemia, eg renal failure or vitamin D deficiency (calcium is low or normal). Tertiary develops in response to secondary hyperparathyroidism and is caused by autonomous parathyroid hyperplasia.

3 J – Multiple myeloma
This man's hypercalcaemia is related to the excessive osteoclast activity caused by the neoplastic clonal proliferation of marrow plasma cells. These abnormal plasma cells produce abnormal immunoglobulins (paraproteins) that may be associated with the excretion of light chains in the urine, which are known as Bence Jones proteins. H. Bence Jones (1814–73) studied medicine at St Georges Hospital, London, and was not only an excellent physician but also a skilled chemist. His insistence of examination of urine both chemically and microscopically was truly ahead of its time. Monoclonal (M) bands on serum protein electrophoresis provide evidence of such proteins and form the cornerstone of diagnosing this condition. Patients present in their 60s with bone pain, anaemia, recurrent infections and bleeding. Renal failure ensues, caused by deposition of light chains in the tubules, hypercalcaemia, hyperuricaemia and amyloid deposition. Paraproteins increase blood viscosity causing blurred vision and gangrene.

90 CAUSES OF SECONDARY HYPERTENSION

In approximately 90% of cases of hypertension no cause can be elucidated and patients are said to have essential hypertension. In the remaining minority an underlying cause can be found, which can be classified into renal, endocrine and miscellaneous, reflecting the control centres of normal blood pressure. An important endocrine pathway to remember is that of the hypothalamic–pituitary–adrenal axis. Corticotrophin-releasing factor (CRF) is produced by the hypothalamus and prompts the pituitary gland to produce adrenocorticotrophic hormone (ACTH). This in turn stimulates the adrenal cortex to produce cortisol, aldosterone and, in smaller amounts, sex hormones. Each of these end-organ hormones feedback in a negative way to the hypothalamus and pituitary gland. Other environmental factors, such as stress, can also stimulate the hypothalamus to release ACTH.

Any young (< 35 years old) patient or individual failing to respond to anti-hypertensive treatment should be screened for secondary causes. Although rare, they are important conditions with surgically correctable outcomes, resulting in a dramatically improved clinical outcome in otherwise pharmaceutically refractory hypertension.

1 L – Phaeochromocytoma

This is a rare (0.1% of hypertension) catecholamine-producing tumour of the sympathetic system (90% are benign). Between 10 and 20% of these tumours are inherited as an autosomal dominant trait, half of these are bilaterally occurring. They can be associated with other tumours such as MEN (multiple endocrine neoplasia) syndromes, neurofibromatosis, von Hippel–Lindau syndrome, Sturge–Weber syndrome and also tuberous sclerosis. Metanephrines (eg vanillomalleic acid or VMA) are the metabolic by-product of normal catecholamine breakdown and 24-h urine collection is used as a screening tool. Diagnosis can be confirmed on plasma measurement of catecholamine, with localisation by computed tomography or metaiodobenzylguanide (MIBG) scan. Treatment is ideally surgical, under α- and β-blockade with phenoxybenzamine and propanolol commenced pre-operatively. These drugs can also be used in patients who are not fit for surgery.

2 M – Polyarteritis nodosa

This systemic condition belongs to the group of vasculitides affecting small to medium-sized arteries. It primarily affects the main visceral arteries with sparing of the pulmonary circulation. It is characterised by a necrotising inflammation of the arterial wall with resultant fibrotic areas on healing and stenosis. It is a disease of young adults, with non-specific symptoms and signs related to the organs involved. The diagnosis is made by biopsy of the affected arterial segments. Left untreated with immunosuppressants, it frequently results in death. A variant of polyarteritis nodosa is Churg–Strauss syndrome, characterised by asthma, intra- and extra-vascular granulomas with splenic and pulmonary vessel involvement, often resulting in infarction.

3 E – Conn's syndrome

Conn's syndrome is a constellation of symptoms resulting from a unilateral adenoma in the adrenal cortex. It accounts for over 75% of hyperaldosteronism, the remainder being related to bilateral adrenocortical hyperplasia and adrenal adenocarcinoma. Unregulated excess aldosterone causes reduced renal losses of sodium and water, and abnormal potassium and hydrogen ion losses. A subsequent increase in circulating volume with a concomitant rise in blood pressure is seen. Negative feedback, via baroreceptors in the juxtaglomerular apparatus, results in low circulating levels of renin and angiotensin. Patients present with hypertension, polyuria, nocturia and polydipsia, muscle cramps, tetany and cardiac arrhythmias related to the resultant hypokalaemic alkalosis. Screening is performed on three separate plasma potassium measurements, and if at least one measurement is < 3.7 mmol/litre then serum aldosterone, renin, angiotensin and urea & electrolytes should be measured again on three separate occasions. Treatment for Conn's syndrome consists of surgical excision following spironolactone 300 mg/24 h for 4 weeks pre-operatively.

4 F – Cushing's syndrome

Cushing's syndrome is caused by persistently and inappropriately elevated adrenal glucocorticoid levels, the many metabolic effects of which are manifested in Cushing's syndrome. Cushing's disease should be distinguished from Cushing's syndrome; the former being a specific reference to excess production of glucocorticoids resulting from inappropriate ACTH secretion from the pituitary. Cushing's syndrome is a general term used to describe all of the abnormalities caused by elevated glucocorticoid production regardless of cause. Cushing's syndrome therefore encompasses both ACTH-dependent and non-independent causes as given below.

ACTH-dependent causes:

- pituitary adenoma (Cushing's disease)
- ectopic ACTH-producing tumours (eg small cell lung carcinoma)

Non-ACTH-dependent causes

- steroid medication
- adrenal tumours/hyperplasia

Vascular surgery

91 THE PAINFUL LOWER LIMB

1 F – Embolus

The scenario describes several of the classic clinical features associated with acute limb ischaemia as a result of arterial embolism (pain, paraesthesia, paralysis, pale, perishing with cold, pulseless). An embolus is the passage of matter from one part of the circulation to another through a vascular lumen. The commonest sources of arterial emboli arise in the heart (thrombus in atrial appendage secondary to atrial fibrillation), from mural thrombus on a myocardial infarct, from aneurysms and atherosclerotic plaques. Peripheral emboli may also arise from the heart valves. Previously, acute endocarditis on a rheumatic heart valve was an important source, but is now rare. More commonly, peripheral emboli occur secondary to acute bacterial endocarditis after intravenous drug abuse with contaminated needles, as in the clinical case described.

2 C – Chronic venous insufficiency

Chronic venous insufficiency describes a spectrum of disease of the lower limb veins in which venous return is chronically impaired by reflux, obstruction, or calf pump failure. This results in sustained venous hypertension, which is associated with clinical complications such as oedema, eczema, lipodermatosclerosis and ulceration. Varicose veins are usually characteristic of this condition, and provide visual confirmation of venous reflux. However, the absence of visible varicose veins does **not** exclude the presence of significant superficial reflux. The pain associated with this condition tends to be worse following prolonged periods of standing (gravitational effects/calf pump not functional), and is relieved by rest and elevation of the affected limb. In the case described (and most commonly) the insufficiency is secondary to previous venous obstruction of the deep veins by thrombosis (DVT).

3 B – Buerger's disease

Buerger's disease (thromboangiitis obliterans) almost exclusively affects young men in their early 20s or 30s who are heavy smokers. It is particularly common in men of Jewish, Arab, Indian and Chinese origin. It has previously been considered as a variant of accelerated atherosclerosis but most now regard it as a separate disease process. It involves progressive obliteration of distal, medium-sized arteries of the lower limb, characterised by transmural round cell infiltration associated with intimal proliferation. Collagen is laid down around the vessels, encasing them in a thick fibrous coat. Patients usually present with distal gangrene, often preceded by a history of claudication. Popliteal pulses are usually preserved, but pedal pulses are absent. Arteriography shows normal proximal vessels and distal occlusions with 'corkscrew' collaterals. Biopsy of the occluded vessel provides histological confirmation of the diagnosis.

92 ULCERATION IN THE LOWER LIMB

1 E – Neuropathic ulcer

These ulcers occur in denervated tissue and result from local ischaemia, usually caused by non-perceived local trauma. They are characteristically painless and have a good blood supply (although diabetic neuropathy being a common cause may also lead to large-vessel atherosclerosis, resulting in a mixed picture of arterial and neuropathic ulceration). The causes of neuropathic ulceration may be divided into peripheral nerve lesions and spinal cord lesions. The former consist of diabetes, nerve injuries and leprosy, while spina bifida, tabes dorsalis and syringomyelia comprise the second group.

2 F – Pyoderma gangrenosum

This man may have undiagnosed ulcerative colitis. The lesions at first resemble boils, which subsequently break down to form necrotic ulcers with purple edges. Pyoderma gangrenosum is also associated with rheumatoid arthritis, multiple myeloma and leukaemia.

3 D – Neoplastic ulcer

This woman has a Marjolin's ulcer or a squamous cell carcinoma arising from chronic inflammation in a long-standing benign ulcer or scar. This commonly occurs in a venous ulcer making constant review of such patients important.

93 THE SWOLLEN LOWER LIMB

Lymphoedema is an accumulation of tissue fluid secondary to a fault in the lymphatic system (abnormalities of lymph formation or lymph clearance). This may be primary, in the absence of other causes, or secondary to malignant disease, surgery (eg post-radical mastectomy/groin dissection), radiotherapy or infection (filariasis, pyogenic tuberculosis). The differential diagnosis of lymphoedema includes other causes of tissue oedema, which may be broadly classified as:

- *systemic disorders, eg cardiac/renal/liver failure, hereditary angio-oedema, etc*
- *venous disorders, eg post-thrombotic syndrome, extrinsic compression (pregnancy/tumour/retroperitoneal fibrosis), Klippel–Trenaunay syndrome*
- *miscellaneous disorders, eg arteriovenous malformations, factitious oedema etc.*

1 A – Angio-oedema

Hereditary angio-oedema is inherited as an autosomal dominant condition. It arises as a result of a deficiency in the complement system regulation, and is characterised by recurrent attacks of swelling of the face and extremities that subsequently resolve. The oedema is often associated with erythema.

2 H – Klippel–Trenaunay syndrome

This syndrome is characterised by dilated veins, associated with bony and soft tissue deformity, elongation of the limb, capillary naevi and limb oedema. There are no arterial abnormalities. The diagnosis is suggested as varicose veins are present since birth or early childhood, and are often present on the outside of the leg, not the inner side where most varicose veins appear.

3 M – Primary lymphoedema

Primary lymphoedema may be classified as:

- congenital – when it occurs soon after birth (and is hereditary in some cases; Milroy's disease)
- praecox – presenting up to the age of 35 years
- tarda – when it presents over the age of 35 years, as in this case.

It has been suggested that these groups represent different parts of the same spectrum of disease, which has been attributed to aplasia, hypoplasia, or hyperplasia of the lymph vessels. Once other causes of oedema have been excluded, the diagnosis of primary lymphoedema may be confirmed using isotope lymphography, computed tomography scanning, magnetic resonance imaging, or contrast lymphangiography. The aims of treatment are to reduce limb swelling and weight, reduce the risk of infection, and improve function. This may be achieved using conservative measures (elevation/compression of affected limb). Surgical intervention involves debulking (of excess skin and subcutaneous tissue) or bypass procedures (where regional blockade of lymphatics is evident).

94 MANAGEMENT OF PERIPHERAL VASCULAR DISORDERS

1 C – Atherosclerosis risk factor reduction

This patient has intermittent claudication, a symptom of chronic lower limb atherosclerosis. Initial management involves: risk factor reduction, including cessation of smoking, lipid-lowering drugs, anti-platelet medication, good diabetic control if appropriate; regular exercise as part of a supervised exercise programme and weight loss. Surgical intervention is only indicated when the patient has disabling claudication, critical limb ischaemia, ulcers, or gangrene. The two main options are: percutaneous angioplasty (preferable) or bypass surgery.

2 N – Surgical thromboembolectomy

This patient has a classic presentation of acute lower ischaemia, with four of the six Ps: pallor, pulselessness, paraesthesia, paralysis, 'perishing' cold and pain. Percutaneous thrombolytic thromboembolectomy is the treatment of choice unless contraindicated, as in this scenario, in which case the patient should procede to surgical thromboembolectomy. Contraindications to thrombolysis include: cerebrovascular accident within the past 2 months, recent surgery, or previous thrombolytic therapy.

3 M – Short saphenous vein surgery

This patient has a classic presentation of symptomatic varicose veins. Injection sclerotherapy is not applicable, first as it is contraindicated in those taking oral contraceptives, and second as it only provides short-term benefit in those with major incompetence of either long or short saphenous veins. The tourniquet test clearly indicates short saphenous incompetence, hence the need for short saphenous ligation and stripping. General consensus would suggest that duplex scanning should be performed to confirm the diagnosis and to site the junction for surgery (this is not necessary for long-saphenous disease unless the veins are recurrent).

Transplant surgery

95 COMPLICATIONS OF CADAVERIC ORGAN TRANSPLANTATION

1 E – Cyclosporin side-effects

Cyclosporin A is an example of a calcineurin inhibitor. Cyclosporin-based triple immunosuppression with corticosteroids and azathioprine remains the most popular regimen in the UK. It is used prophylactically and therapeutically to address rejection following organ transplantation. Side-effects of cyclosporin include nephrotoxicity, hypertension, hirsutism, tremor, gingival hyperplasia and hepatotoxicity. Long-term use increases the risk of development of malignancy (5% of patients), most commonly basal or squamous cell carcinomas.

2 F – Cytomegalovirus infection

In addition to the development of malignancy, immunosuppression increases the risk of infection. Cytomegalovirus (CMV) is a member of the herpes group of viruses. Primary infection in a seronegative individual who receives a graft from a seropositive donor typically occurs 6 weeks post-transplantation, and results in the most severe disease. The main symptoms of CMV infection are usually non-specific and include fever, night sweats, fatigue and myalgia. Retinitis is pathognomonic, but rarely seen in the transplant population. Respiratory distress, noticed at first during exercise, may give a clue to early CMV pneumonitis. Patients may also present with CMV encephalitis or gastrointestinal infection, characterised by dysphagia, diarrhoea, nausea and abdominal pain. Reactivation of latent CMV infection may also occur in immunosuppressed patients, although the infection is usually less severe.

3 D – Chronic rejection

Chronic rejection is characterised clinically by a progressive deterioration in graft function occurring months to years after transplantation and is associated with typical histological changes of graft atherosclerosis and fibrosis. By contrast, acute rejection occurs within the first 3 months after transplantation, and hyperacute rejection occurs within hours. For the diagnosis of chronic rejection to be made, other causes of graft dysfunction must be excluded (eg infection, calcineurin antagonist toxicity, etc), and a transplant graft biopsy is required to confirm the diagnosis histologically. For renal transplantation, graft dysfunction is manifested by a rise in serum creatinine as a result of progressive decline in the glomerular filtration rate. There is associated proteinuria and worsening hypertension, with the diastolic component classically rising in advance of the systolic component.

Ear, nose and throat, and maxillofacial surgery

96 AUDITORY DISORDERS

1 K – Ménière's disease

Prosper Ménière (1799–1862) was a French ENT specialist, assistant of Baron Dupuytren and friend of Balzac and Victor Hugo. The condition he described is characterised by deafness, dizziness and tinnitus (or din), ie the three Ds (as in this patient). All patients presenting with vertigo should have imaging to exclude an acoustic neuroma (this diagnosis would be more strongly suspected if evidence of cranial nerve/cerebellar dysfunction coexisted), and testing for syphilis, as neurosyphilis may present in this way and must be treated.

2 F – Cholesteotoma

This is a form of chronic suppurative otitis media. As a result of a marginal or attic perforation, there is chronic infection of the bone of the attic, antrum and mastoid process, as well as the mucosa of the middle ear. While the disease is less common than in pre-antibiotic times, it is an important disorder not to miss. Cholesteotoma requires chronic treatment, often including surgery (commonly mastoidectomy) and has numerous potentially serious extra- and intra-cranial complications.

3 M – Otosclerosis

This common disorder occurs in approximately 1/200 people to some degree. The disorder is more common in women, and has a marked hereditary tendency in certain families. It commonly presents between the ages of 18 and 30. The pathology is one of excessive bone formation in the middle ear that leads to conductive deafness, hence the findings on Rinne's (negative when bone conduction is superior to air) and Weber's tests (lateralises to worse side) and often also tinnitus. The hearing is often improved in noisy places: so-called paracusis Willisii. The tympanum appears normal in the majority of cases.

4 C – Acute suppurative otitis media

The taxonomy in this area is rather confusing, there being a variety of middle ear effusions described in terms of their duration (acute versus chronic), the presence or absence of infection (unspecified = serous versus suppurative), as well as other factors such as their aetiology, eg acute catarrhal otitis media (a variant of acute serous) and the use of popular terms such as glue ear (chronic serous). In terms of examination, the tympanic membrane is retracted in all except acute suppurative, where it is bulging, and chronic suppurative, where it is nearly always perforated (this being the aetiology of the chronic infection).

97 EPISTAXIS

The commonest causes of epistaxis are: idiopathic (nose picking), external trauma and rhinitis (allergic and infective). Other causes may also be local or secondary to systemic disease (especially blood dyscrasias). Iatrogenic causes include anticoagulant therapy and nasogastric tubes.

1 B – Foreign body

This may present with bleeding from the nose in the presence of long-standing inflammation. The history of a foul-smelling nasal discharge and the age of the child (foreign bodies in the nose are commonest in children aged 2–3) should alert one to the diagnosis. Treatment is by removal under general anaesthesia once inflammation is established as in this case. If the problem is identified early, various manoeuvres can be attempted in The Emergency Department to blow out the offending foreign body.

2 A – Chemical irritation

In this case, the patient is likely to be a regular user of cocaine (now one of the most common causes of recurrent epistaxis). The diagnosis is strongly suggested by the septal defect, dental problems and sinus problems, especially in a young adult.

98 VOCAL PROBLEMS: DYSPHONIA

Dysphonia is defined as an impairment of voice, and can be divided into two categories:

- *problems with projection of voice*
- *problems with quality of voice.*

The commonest of the latter is hoarseness, a form of dysphonia defined as a rough or noisy quality of voice. However, hoarseness is often used interchangeably with dysphonia. Broadly speaking, the causes of dysphonia may be divided into those leading to damage in some way to the mucosal surfaces of the cords, eg inflammation, tumour, and those leading to vocal cord paralysis.

1 C – Gastro-oesophageal reflux disease (GORD)

This is suggested by early diurnal hoarseness and the absence of any evident pathology on indirect laryngoscopy. It is one example of non-infectious inflammatory changes of the vocal cords, sometimes referred to as chronic laryngitis. The other common causes are chronic cough and heavy smoking.

2 G – Neurogenic: Left recurrent laryngeal nerve palsy

In this case this has arisen as a result of carcinoma of the left bronchus (see other symptoms and signs). Vocal cord paralysis arises as a rule from remote causes and the causes vary bilaterally as a result of differences in the anatomical course of the recurrent laryngeal nerve on each side. On the left the student will recall that the nerve loops around the remnant of the ductus arteriosus (so passing below the arch of the aorta versus the subclavian artery on the right). This makes it susceptible to left hilar pathologies (tumours, pulmonary surgery, left atrial enlargement etc). The cord lies in the paramedian (adducted) position in contrast to lesions of the vagus or superior laryngeal nerves in which it lies in the cadaveric (abducted) position, usually causing aphonia.

3 F – Laryngeal papilloma

These are viral lesions that commonly arise between the ages of 2 and 5 years. They must be removed with care, as they can easily be spread to the whole of the larynx and trachea. Laser removal, which vaporises the lesions, is the treatment of choice. They are said to disappear at puberty although this is the exception rather than the rule. Multiple papillomas are a cause of stridor and respiratory obstruction, sometimes necessitating tracheostomy.

99 STRIDOR

1 B – Acute laryngotracheobronchitis

This condition, also referred to as 'croup', is caused by viral infection (parainfluenza 1) and commonly affects the 6-month to 3-year-old age group in the winter months. The stridor (and sometimes respiratory obstruction) is caused by subglottic oedema. Treatment is with humidified air/oxygen in an incubator (or croupette) to prevent crusting, intravenous antibiotics and supportive intravenous fluids. Scrupulous observation is required for signs of impending respiratory obstruction that would require nasotracheal intubation by a skilled anaesthetist or tracheostomy (if this fails). The condition is distinguished from acute epiglottitis, where the child is usually older, and the presence of supraglottic oedema (the epiglottis is red and swollen and protrudes above the tongue: the rising sun sign). Diphtheria is a differential diagnosis in unimmunised populations.

2 D – Angioneurotic oedema

This is a condition of unknown aetiology most commonly affecting young women. Management is by close observation, antihistamines and intravenous steroids/epinephrine nebulisers. Should the condition deteriorate, the patient may require orotracheal intubation. It is distinguished only from anaphylactic shock by the absence of a precipitating allergen (antibiotics/bee stings etc).

3 J – Inhalation or ingestion of irritants

In this case the patient has smoke inhalation with burns to the upper airway. The supraglottic airway is extremely susceptible to obstruction as a result of exposure to heat. When a patient is admitted to hospital after burn injury you must always be alert to the possibility of airway involvement. Clinical indications of inhalation injury include facial burns, singeing of the nasal hairs, carbon deposits in the oropharynx, carbonaceous sputum, hoarseness and a carboxyhaemoglobin level > 10%. The symptom of stridor is an indication for immediate orotracheal intubation, although one should hopefully have electively intubated the patient before this sign is present. A similar pattern of airway obstruction can be causes by ingestion of corrosives such as strong acids and alkalis.

100 NON-NEOPLASTIC SALIVARY GLAND DISEASE

1 E – Sialolithiasis

Calculi can occur in the submandibular or parotid glands, although the former is most commonly affected. Predisposing factors include chronic sialadenitis, reduced salivary flow rates, dehydration and duct obstruction. Calculi are associated with diabetes mellitus, hypertension and chronic liver disease. A stone within a gland may be asymptomatic, whereas a stone in the duct is likely to cause painful swelling that is precipitated by eating. Acute suppurative sialadenitis may supervene, and this is characterised by fever and severe pain that may give rise to spasm of the adjacent muscles of mastication, leading to ' trismus'; such a patient may be toxic. Twenty per cent of submandibular, and 66% of parotid, calculi are radiolucent, and so sialography is indicated to demonstrate filling defects. Stones may be removed surgically by lithotomy (distal stones) or excision of the duct with the gland (proximal stones).

2 F – Sialosis

Sialosis refers to recurrent swelling of the salivary glands in the absence of neoplasia or inflammation. The swelling is typically painless and bilateral. An important distinguishing feature from other causes of parotidomegaly is the fact that the gland, although enlarged, remains soft and not indurated. Sialosis occurs in association with endocrine disorders (myxoedema, Cushing's disease, diabetes mellitus etc), metabolic disturbances (nutritional disorders, vitamin deficiencies etc), and certain drugs [eg dextropropoxyphene (co-proxamol), oral contraceptives, anti-psychotics, clonidine etc].

3 G – Sjögren's syndrome

The salivary glands may be damaged by autoimmune disease. Sjögren's syndrome is characterised by the presence of two of the following triad: keratoconjunctivitis sicca (dry eyes); xerostomia (dry mouth); and rheumatoid arthritis or other connective tissue disorder (eg scleroderma, systemic lupus erythematosus, polyarteritis nodosa etc). The clinical scenario presented describes a patient with primary Sjögren's syndrome, which consists of xerostomia and xerophthalmia, with no connective tissue component. By contrast, secondary Sjögren's syndrome refers to the presence of all three features. The main differential in 'at risk' groups is that of human immunodeficiency virus-associated sialadenitis, which is clinically indistinguishable. This diagnosis should be considered, especially in female patients because Sjögren's has a 10 : 1 female predominance. Mikulicz's syndrome is also an autoimmune syndrome that describes enlargement of the salivary glands, xerostomia and enlargement of the lacrimal glands that cause a bulge below the outer end of the eyelids, and a narrowing in the palpebral fissures.

101 SALIVARY GLAND TUMOURS

1 I – Pleomorphic adenoma

This tumour is a slow-growing lesion that is made up of glandular and stromal elements. It does not have a true capsule but a pseudo-capsule resulting from fibrosis of the adjacent compressed salivary tissue. Multiple projections extending through 'defects' in the pseudo-capsule into the normal surrounding gland prevent its treatment by enucleation. Clinically, pleomorphic adenomas present as slow-growing painless masses. There is rarely disruption of the facial nerve, although location in the deep part of the gland may displace adjacent structures inside the mouth. The diagnosis is confirmed by fine-needle aspiration. Such tumours should be removed by superficial parotidectomy when the tumour is in the superficial lobe of the gland, or by total parotidectomy with preservation of the facial nerve in those tumours involving the deep part of the gland. Those arising in the submandibular gland should be treated by excision of the gland.

2 H – Mucoepidermoid carcinoma

This is the most common malignant salivary gland tumour. Associated pain is not a reliable indicator of malignancy but it is associated with a worse prognosis in proven malignancy. Presentation with facial nerve palsy is very suggestive of a malignant tumour. Twenty-five per cent of patients have associated lymphadenopathy at the time of presentation. Histologically, the tumour is composed of epidermoid cells and mucous cells, which secrete mucus into the stroma of the tumour, giving rise to its cystic nature. Tumours may be graded as high- or low-grade, although their biological behaviour tends to be unpredictable. The 10-year survival rates are 40% and 80% for high-grade and low-grade tumours, respectively.

3 E – Lymphoma

Primary salivary gland lymphomas are uncommon, accounting for 10% of all salivary malignancies. The majority tend to be non-Hodgkin's lymphoma. Patients with non-Hodgkin's usually present with localised or generalised non-tender lymphadenopathy. Approximately 40% of patients have bone marrow involvement at presentation, resulting in cytopenia. There may be associated splenic or hepatic enlargement.

102 NECK LUMPS

When considering neck lumps, it may be helpful to consider the anatomy of the neck and its sub-division into the anterior and posterior triangles. However, it is the Editor's view that, in practice, there is a broad division into three:

- *lymphadenopathy (cervical or supraclavicular) – at the side and common*
- *thyroid lumps/enlargement (and thyroid gland cyst) – in the middle and common*
- *oddities (many of which are embryologic) – at the side and rare.*

1 A – Branchial cyst

A branchial cyst is a remnant of, usually, the second branchial cleft. It is lined by squamous epithelium and if infected, a small sinus may develop tracking to the skin at the anterior border of the sternocleidomastoid muscle. Presentation is often as in the scenario, with the cyst arising from the junction between the upper and middle thirds of the sternocleidomastoid muscle. Treatment is surgical excision with concomitant antibiotic treatment of any pre-existing infection. Care must be taken to excise the entire cyst to prevent recurrence but it is not necessary to trace and excise any tract to the pharynx. Patients must be made fully aware of and give full consent regarding the risks of damage to the accessory, vagus and hypoglossal nerves. Rarely a chronically infected cyst may become adherent to the internal jugular vein.

2 F – Pharyngeal pouch

Also known as Zenker's diverticulum, pharyngeal pouches often present in the elderly where they have had opportunity to develop without many symptoms. Patients eventually complain as in this scenario with dysphagia and subsequent weight loss. Pulmonary overspill occurs and hoarseness and recurrent chest infections may be the only presenting feature. A low, anterior triangular mass may be felt and fluid within the pouch can sometimes be displaced on deeper palpation. Their aetiology is unknown but imaging studies have suggested a neuromuscular inco-ordination resulting in herniation of the mucosa through the muscular coat. The weakest point is Killian's dehiscence between the thyropharyngeal and cricopharyngeal muscles that constitute the inferior constrictor muscle. Management involves surgical excision using an open or endoscopic technique where appropriate.

3 G – Sternocleidomastoid tumour

These appear 1–2 months after birth and are usually accompanied by a history of a complicated or breech birth. The 'tumour' is unilateral and situated as described in this scenario. It is initially a haematoma with associated muscle degeneration. It is often tender at first and associated with a torticollis. Early treatment is imperative, to prevent permanent disability, with active stimulation and passive stimulation which can be achieved at home by the infant's parents. This normally reduces the 'tumour' over the first 4–6 months. Only those that are noted late or fail to respond to conservative treatment require surgery.

4 I – Thyroglossal cyst

In the embryo, the thyroid gland develops from the thyroglossal duct that originates at the foramen caecum at the base of the tongue. Occasionally the duct may remain patent and a structure known as a thyroglossal cyst can persist. These cysts are the commonest midline neck masses of infancy, and may be confused with epidermoid cysts, dermoid cysts and pyramidal lobe thyroid nodules. They are lined with squamous or ciliated pseudo-stratified columnar epithelium. Occasionally they contain lymphoid or thyroid tissue, and any of its constituents may undergo malignant change. Management involves surgical excision of the cyst and the central portion of the hyoid bone in a procedure known as Sistrunk's operation, to ensure that the condition does not recur.

103 ORAL/GLOSSAL LESIONS

1 E – Pyogenic granuloma

The history of trauma (in this case secondary to the use of the mouth-piece of breathing apparatus) and rapid growth are characteristic of this condition. There is an overgrowth of granulation tissue, which gives rise to a 'nodular' lesion that may bleed or produce serous or purulent fluid. Excision biopsy is necessary to confirm the diagnosis histologically.

2 F – Ranula

A ranula is a large mucus-containing cyst in the floor of the mouth. *Ranula* is Latin for a small frog, as the swelling is said to resemble the 'belly of a frog'. A ranula develops on one side of the floor of the mouth, and slowly enlarges to form a bluish fluctuant swelling beneath the sublingual mucosa that transilluminates. The cysts have thin walls and easily rupture. Treatment is by surgical excision, with care to avoid injury to the submandibular duct or lingual nerve.

3 A – Carcinoma of the oral cavity

Squamous cell carcinoma is the principal cancer of the oral cavity. Aetiological factors include excessive **S**moking and alcohol consumption (**S**pirits), which have a synergistic effect on risk. A range of other factors, including **S**yphilis, papillomavirus infection and repeated trauma (**S**ore tooth), are suggested in the aetiology, although causative evidence is lacking. The most common presenting features are ulceration, pain, swelling and a neck lump. Tumours metastasise to the cervical lymph nodes. Synchronous and metachronous tumours occur in 5% and 10%, respectively. Surgery and/or radiotherapy are the mainstays of treatment, the decision being based on the location and size of tumour.

104 CERVICAL LYMPHADENOPATHY

The causes of cervical lymphadenopathy can be classified into four groups:

- *primary malignancy (lymphomas and leukaemias, ie lymphoreticular disease)*
- *metastatic malignancy (local carcinomas)*
- *infections*
- *sarcoid*

1 D – Metastatic malignancy

This position describes that of the cervical lymph nodes that drain the oropharynx and larynx. The lymphatic system of the neck can be divided into Levels 1–5. This man has palpable Level 3 nodes that also drain Levels 1 and 2, which receive lymph from the scalp, face and lips. The most likely diagnosis here is a laryngeal carcinoma given the dysphonia.

2 G – Tonsillitis

This acute history and anatomical description of involved lymph nodes is typical of tonsillitis, remembering that the tonsil itself is a lymphoid structure. Other acute causes of cervical lymphadenopathy include pharyngitis/laryngitis and Epstein–Barr virus infection. Chronic causes include tuberculosis and sarcoidosis.

3 C – Lymphoreticular disease

This is fairly obvious given the history. The differential would be tuberculosis/human immunodeficiency virus in at-risk individuals.

Paediatric surgery

105 PAEDIATRIC SURGICAL DISORDERS

1 J – Meconeum ileus

The sweat test provides a definitive diagnosis of cystic fibrosis, although this can be confirmed by gene probe which demonstrates the mutation on the long arm of chromosome 7. Around 10–15% of affected infants present at birth with meconium ileus. Obstruction is caused by thick, sticky meconium within the distal ileum lumen. Diagnosis is suspected on plain abdominal radiograph, which shows dilated loops of bowel, absence of air-fluid levels and a 'soap bubble' appearance in the right lower quadrant. If uncomplicated, the obstruction may be relieved by a therapeutic gastrograffin enema (hyperosmolar and emulsifying action); the success rate is approximately 55%. If unsuccessful, infants require an enterotomy and mechanical washout.

2 K – Necrotising enterocolitis

This predominantly affects pre-term infants, and is one of the commonest surgical emergencies in the neonatal period. Pathogenesis involves intestinal ischaemia, bacterial colonisation and translocation, and presence of milk formula in the intestinal lumen. The radiological finding of intramural gas, (pneumatosis intestinalis), is pathognomonic. Management involves nasogastric decompression, broad-spectrum antibiotics, fluid resuscitation and parenteral nutrition; it is successful in 70–80% of cases.

3 H – Intussusception

This is the most common cause of abdominal emergency in infants between 3 and 24 months, with incidence peaking at 6–9 months. Most cases are idiopathic, the intussusceptum being an enlarged Peyer's patch secondary to a viral infection. The intussusceptum invaginates into neighbouring bowel, (the intussuscipiens), causing subacute intestinal obstruction and venous compression of the intussusceptum. The diagnosis may be made on the classical clinical findings of intermittent, recurrent attacks of screaming and the infant drawing up its knees, passage of blood per rectum and a palpable sausage-shaped mass. Diagnosis may be confirmed by contrast enema or ultrasound scan. Reduction, by air or contrast enema under fluoroscopic or ultrasound control, can be successful in up to 90% of infants.

4 L – Pyloric stenosis

This occurs most commonly at 4–6 weeks of age and typically presents with projectile non-bilious vomiting. Diagnosis is usually made by palpation of an 'olive-shaped' mass in the right hypochondrium. If in doubt, ultrasound is the investigation of choice. Management involves fluid resuscitation and a pyloromyotomy, which can be performed as open surgery or laparoscopically.

Plastic surgery

106 MANAGEMENT OF BURNS

The answers to this question rely on the candidate's specific knowledge of two areas of burn management: the fluid calculation formula (below) and the American Burn Association guidelines for transfer to a burn centre (both contained within the ATLS student manual – with which you should be familiar).

Formula = 2–4 ml Ringer's lactate/kg/% BSA partial or full-thickness burn over 24 h; 50% given in the first 8 hours and 50% in the second 16 hours.

1 C – 1–2 litres Ringer's lactate solution in 8 h

By calculation: 2–4 ml × 70 × 14 = 2–4 litres over 24 h; ie 1–2 litres over first 8 h. The patient does not meet the guidelines for transfer, these are (for an adult) > 20% BSA total burns (second or third degree) or > 5% full-thickness (third degree) burns. Other criteria for transfer in an adult include injuries to specific body areas, eg eyes, ears, face, hands, genitalia, associated inhalation injury, and specific types of burn, eg electrical/certain chemical.

2 B – 0.5–1 litres Ringer's lactate solution in 8 h, transfer to burns unit

By calculation: 2–4 ml × 35 × 14 = 1–2 litres over 24 h; ie 0.5–1 litres over first 8 h. Any child (< 10 years) with partial or full-thickness burns affecting > 10% BSA should be referred to a burns unit.

3 H – 4–8 litres Ringer's lactate solution in 8 h, transfer to burns unit

This requires one more mental step – that of knowing the 'Rule of Nines' used to calculate BSA affected by burns (also in the ATLS handbook). The front and back of the trunk are 18% each and the front and back of a lower limb are 9% (for completion, the front and back of the upper limbs and head are 4.5% each). Therefore, by calculation he has (18 × 2) + (9 × 2) = 54%

burns. So his fluid requirement is 2–4 ml × 70 × 54 = 8–16 litres (to one significant figure) over 24 h; ie 4–8 litres over first 8 h. The patient clearly requires transfer.

107 BENIGN SKIN AND SUBCUTANEOUS LESIONS

1 E – Ganglion

A ganglion is a cystic, myxomatous degeneration of fibrous tissue. They can occur anywhere but are commonly found over the dorsum of the hand over the scapholunate ligament. They are most evident when the wrist is flexed and commonly occur in people handling heavy objects or who traumatise the hand. Some reduce on movement of the joint but they are not truly emptying into a joint space. They can be uncomfortable and cosmetically unsightly. Resection of part of the sac can be performed but recurrence may be as high as 20%. A differential diagnosis includes a bursa or a mucous cyst, the latter caused by a 'blow-out' of an osteoarthritic joint.

2 H – Keratoacanthoma

This benign lesion is a rapidly growing collection of hair follicle cells, that is self-limiting and often regresses leaving a small puckered scar. It can be mistaken for a basal cell carcinoma, although it tends to be perfectly round, and histologically can resemble a small cell carcinoma. The lesion consists of normal skin with a central necrotic or keratinous core. There is never any extension into local tissues and local lymph nodes should not be involved. Treatment is usually expectant for a short time because they can resolve. However, if in doubt then there is case for early removal to exclude malignancy as well as for cosmetic reasons.

3 J – Lymphangioma circumscriptum

This is a collection of dilated lymph sacs in the skin and subcutaneous tissue that fail to drain into the normal lymphatic system. Larger cysts found purely in the subcutaneous tissue are known as cystic hygromas. They are of unknown aetiology but are probably an aberrant developmental condition where these vesicles fail to connect to draining lymph structures. They tend to occur at the junction between the limbs and neck with the trunk. Commonly found in children, they often present because parents notice the vesicles when they become blood-filled, subsequently causing them to become bloodstained, brown or black in colour as the blood becomes haemolysed.

4 M – Pyogenic granuloma

This lesion is a benign reactive inflammatory mass produced in response to trauma, composed of granulation tissue and blood vessels. They erupt rapidly and have a polypoid appearance and a 'collar' around the base. Profuse contact bleeding is often a presenting symptom. They should be differentiated from a squamous cell carcinoma, amelanotic melanoma and Kaposi's sarcoma. Treatment involves curettage or excision followed by histological examination.

108 PIGMENTED LESIONS OF THE SKIN

1 G – Deep capillary naevus

These are also known as port-wine stains and are formed by capillaries in the upper and deeper dermis. Together with superficial capillary naevi ('stork marks'), it belongs to the group of vascular naevi. Most occur on the head and neck and tend to be unilateral, often appearing in the territory of one or more branches of the trigeminal nerve. They can be extensive and cosmetically disfiguring. At birth they can vary from pink to dark purple, darkening over time. Lumpy angiomatous nodules may also develop within the lesion. Often these lesions can be lasered with reasonable results. There are some important considerations:

- associated intracranial vascular malformation resulting in convulsions and delayed development, known as Sturge–Weber syndrome
- congenital glaucoma if lesion occurs in ophthalmic division of trigeminal nerve
- hypertrophy of underlying tissues, eg the limb, causing abnormal growth known as haemangiectatic hypertrophy.

2 O – Strawberry naevus

These lesions appear shortly after birth and tend to occur around the head, neck and napkin area. The lesion can grow rapidly to produce a dome-shaped, red-purple extrusion which can be friable. Despite being unsightly, they usually undergo spontaneous resolution, beginning with an alarming-looking area of central necrosis. Generally, 50% regress by the age of 5 years and 70% by the age of 7 years. Therefore management is expectant but there are specific indications for surgery such as breathing/feeding difficulties or haemorrhage. Medical treatment is high-dose prednisolone but in more severe cases, complex surgical intervention may be required.

3 K – Lentigo

This man has Peutz–Jeghers syndrome, which is an autosomal condition consisting of hamartomatous polyps of the small and large bowel and melanotic pigmentation as described in the scenario. There is also an increased risk of carcinoma of the pancreas, breast, lung, ovary and uterus. A lentigo is a pigmented lesion that consists of excess melanocytes in a normal position, ie above the dermis, producing a normal amount of melanin. This compares with a freckle, which is composed of a normal quantity of melanocytes in a normal position producing excess melanin. A mole or pigmented naevus has excess melanocytes in clusters producing excess melanin. Depending on the location of these clusters with respect to the dermis, these can be described as intradermal, compound, or junctional.

4 Q – Superficial spreading melanoma

This is the commonest type of melanoma in the UK and this woman's lesion is typical of this type of melanoma, which has a radial growth phase before true invasion begins. Clinically, there is an irregularly pigmented patch with an irregular edge. The lesion may itch, give discomfort, or bleed. They tend to occur on the legs and arms in women and the trunk region on men.

109 MALIGNANT MELANOMA

The revised American Joint Committee on Cancer (AJCC) staging sytem for cutaneous malignancy is the most commonly used method. Initial classification is according to Tumour, Nodes and Metastases (ie TNM). The TNM classification is then used to stage the disease from stage 0 to IV. The system is summarised below (subscript a indicates without ulceration, subscript b indicates with ulceration).

<u>T classification</u>

- T_{is} – *malignant melanoma* in situ
- T_1 – ≤ *1.00 mm*
- T_2 – *1.01–2.00 mm*
- T_3 – *2.01–4.0 mm*
- T_4 – > *4.0 mm*

<u>N classification</u>

- N_0 – *no lymph node involvement*
- N_1 – *one lymph node*
- N_2 – *two or three lymph nodes, or satellite/in-transit lesions*
- N_3 – *four or more lymph nodes*

<u>M classification</u>

- M_0 – *no metastases*
- M_{1a} – *distant skin or lymph node metastases*
- M_{1b} – *lung metastases*
- M_{1c} – *all other visceral metastases*

<u>Stage</u>

- *0* – T_{is}, N_0, M_0
- *I* – T_{1a}–T_{2a}, N_0, M_0
- *II* – T_{2b}–T_{4b}, N_0, M_0
- *III – Any T*, N_{1-3}, M_0
- *IV – Any T, any N*, M_{1a-c}

In accordance with this system the answers are:

1 F – T_{2b} lesion

This is indicated by the thickness of the lesion and the presence of ulceration. No comment is made on lymph node status.

2 B – Stage III disease

This patient has metastatic disease to his regional lymph nodes without any evidence of distant spread, hence stage III. This is regardless of the thickness of the primary and the number of lymph nodes affected. He would be N_2 or N_3 depending on the number of nodes affected.

3 C – Stage IV disease

This patient has stage IV disease based on the clinical finding of visceral metastases (irregular hepatomegaly). In addition there is also a suspicion of pulmonary metastases. This, of course, would need confirmation by means of staging investigations.

110 SKIN ULCERS

Ulcers are correctly described (as in this question) in terms of their location, size, shape, edge, base and discharge; a point that should be remembered by the candidate throughout the examination. The other most favoured examiner's question is probably the definition which is: 'a discontinuation of an epithelial surface'.

1 C – Chancrous ulcer (syphilitic chancre)

The classic description, site and short duration after unprotected sex, makes this a strong possibility. Classically termed a Hunterian chancre (presumably by first description rather than first-hand experience), this is the pathognomic lesion of primary syphilis. The other ulcer in syphilis, a gummatous ulcer, occurs as a late manifestation of the infection at a site distant from that of sexual contact and as a result of a granulomatous hypersensitivity reaction.

2 A – Anthrax

Caused by the large Gram-positive aerobic spore-forming organism *Bacillus anthracis,* this is the description of cutaneous anthrax (the most common type). The organism is found in cattle and so those affected are usually dairy or beef farmers, zookeepers, cowboys and buffalo hunters. Inhaled and swallowed spores may result in acute shortness of breath (pulmonary anthrax) and gastrointestinal bleeding (gastrointestinal anthrax). Treatment is with parenteral penicillin.

Neurosurgery

111 HEAD INJURY (TYPES)

1 A – Basal skull fracture

Skull fractures may be of the vault or base. Basal skull fractures usually require computed tomography (CT) scanning (bone windows) for identification. The clinical signs include, however, 'racoon' or 'panda' eyes (as in this case), retroauricular eccymosis (ie mastoid bruising = Battle's sign), subconjunctival haemorrhage and blood in the external auditory meatus. Such fractures rarely require intervention but may be associated with cerebrospinal fluid leaks from ear or nose, or with cranial nerve palsies (as well as neurological injury). All should have 24-h neurological observation. Antibiotics are not now administered.

2 H – Le Fort II fracture

Much of the understanding of patterns of fracture propagation in midface trauma originates from the work of René Le Fort. In 1901, his work on cadaver skulls that were subjected to blunt forces of various magnitudes and directions demonstrated that predictable patterns of fractures follow certain types of injuries. Three predominant types were described which roughly correlate with increasing severity of injury, especially in terms of associated brain injury. Fractures can be uni- or bilateral. The classification is a slight simplification because, in practice, combinations occur, however, it remains useful. Briefly (although best seen pictorially): a Le Fort I (horizontal) fracture extends from the nasal septum laterally through the maxilla just above the teeth and thence backwards to the pterygoid region; a Le Fort II (pyramidal) fracture is as described here; and a Le Fort III (transverse) fracture is an anatomically complex injury which is often bilateral and which extends right across the frontoethmoid regions, superior and lateral orbits to the zygomatic arch laterally and back through the ethmoid to the sphenoid. It is a form of craniofacial dysjunction.

3 C – Diffuse axonal injury

This is the most severe type of diffuse brain injury (less severe are defined as mild concussion and classic cerebral concussion). There is no focal injury requiring emergency evacuation. The appearances are those of cerebral oedema and raised intracranial pressure. Treatment should be aimed at medically reducing intracranial pressure (< 25 mmHg) and increasing cerebral perfusion pressure and oxygenation. The prognosis is very poor.

4 D – Extradural haematoma

These are located outside the dura but within the skull. They are most commonly located in and associated with injuries of the temporal or temporoparietal region and often result from tearing of the middle meningeal artery by a fracture. Because they are commonly not associated with primary brain injury, there is classically a 'lucid interval' before a rapid decline in neurological status as a result of cerebral compression from arterial bleeding. The so-called 'talk and die' scenario.

112 HEAD INJURY (GLASGOW COMA SCALE)

In clinical practice you have the observation chart in front of you. In College examinations regrettably you do not!

1 D – GCS 7

E = 2, M = 3, V = 2.

2 I – GCS 12

E = 3, M = 5, V = 4.

3 F – GCS 9

E = 2, M = 4, V = 3.

113 MANAGEMENT OPTIONS IN A PATIENT WITH HEAD INJURY

The primary aim of clinical and radiological assessment of patients with head injury is to identify those patients with clinically important brain injury and, most crucially, those with an intracranial haematoma requiring urgent neurosurgical management. The vast majority of head injuries are classified as 'mild' with a low-risk of intracranial haematoma. Previously, skull X-ray has been heavily relied upon to triage patients with mild head injury but the sensitivity of this investigation may be as low as 38%. Therefore, it is currently only justified if computed tomography (CT) is not available, or when non-accidental injury in children is suspected. By contrast, CT scanning has a sensitivity and specificity approaching 100%, and so the Royal College of Surgeons Guidelines state that 24-h CT is required in all centres receiving head-injured patients.

1 C – CT scan

Despite the apparently trivial mechanism of injury and the normal Glasgow Coma Scale (GCS), this lady has two clinical features that indicate risk of a clinically significant brain injury (age > 64 years and more than one episode of vomiting). The Canadian Head CT Rule was derived from a cohort of more than 3000 patients using multivariate analysis of several risk factors, and has identified the following clinical features that indicate that there is a clinically significant brain injury requiring neurosurgical intervention:

- GCS < 13 at any point since injury
- GCS 13 or 14 with failure to regain GCS 15 within 2 h
- suspected open or depressed skull fracture
- any sign of basal skull fracture (Battle's sign, haemotympanum etc)
- more than one episode of vomiting
- age > 64 years
- post-traumatic seizure
- coagulopathy (including anti-coagulant therapy)
- focal neurological deficit.

CT scan should be performed within 1 h in all such patients. Two further features in the absence of the above indicate a risk of clinically significant brain injury that does not require neurosurgical intervention: retrograde amnesia of > 30 min and dangerous mechanism of injury (pedestrian hit by vehicle, fall from a height etc). CT scan in such patients may be delayed for up to 8 h.

2 E – Discharge and head injury instructions

Patients with trivial head injury, and who are fully orientated, have no history of loss of consciousness or amnesia, nor any other clinical risk factors, as described above, have a negligible risk of a clinically important brain injury and do not require imaging. The risk of complications requiring hospital care is low enough to warrant discharge to the care of a responsible adult with head injury instructions. All patients with a head injury must receive such instructions before discharge. Similarly, patients with a normal CT scan and no other social or clinical risk factors may be discharged with head injury instructions.

3 I – Endotracheal intubation

This patient has several risk factors for significant brain injury requiring urgent neurosurgical intervention. Clearly, he requires a CT scan, but this is currently unavailable in the receiving Unit. A skull X-ray is unlikely to provide sufficient information relating to the degree of brain injury sustained, and therefore this patient should be transferred to a Neurosurgical Unit where clinical and radiological assessment may be performed. In addition, there is a clear indication to administer an intravenous bolus of mannitol (1 g /kg) in this case, because there is a history of deterioration in consciousness level and pupil changes, secondary to rising intracranial pressure. The creation of an emergency burr hole performed by a general surgeon is not generally recommended or supported, and can only be justified in patients with rapidly expanding intracranial haematomas that are imminently life-threatening, and when definitive neurosurgical care is unavailable. Neither criteria are met, as the diagnosis is not yet clear, and neurosurgical care is available. However, before mannitol and transfer (which you might have been tempted to choose), he will require intubation, 'A' being before 'D'.

114 SPINAL CORD INJURY

1 G – Neurogenic shock

Neurogenic shock results from impairment of the descending sympathetic pathways in the spinal cord. It usually results from cervical, or 'high' thoracic spinal cord injury. Loss of sympathetic innervation results in loss of vasomotor tone, and sympathetic innervation to the heart. Consequently, there is vasodilatation, pooling of blood in the extremities, and hence hypotension. In addition, there may be evidence of bradycardia, or at least failure of the sympathetic-driven tachycardia in response to hypovolaemia. The hypotension is not normalised by fluid resuscitation but may respond to the judicious use of vasopressors. Atropine may be used to address the bradycardia. By contrast, spinal shock refers to the flaccidity and loss of reflexes seen after spinal cord injury.

2 F – Incomplete spinal injury

In addition to the level of neurological deficit, the severity is also important. Such injuries may be classified as complete or incomplete. Any motor or sensory function below the level of the injury constitutes an incomplete injury. An incomplete injury may be suggested by the presence of sacral sparing. This involves preservation of peri-anal sensation, voluntary anal sphincter contraction, or voluntary toe flexion. However, preservation of spinal reflexes (eg bulbocavernosus, anal wink, or deep tendon reflexes) alone does not qualify as an incomplete injury.

3 C – Central cord syndrome

Certain characteristic clinical patterns of incomplete neurological injury may be recognised. Central cord syndrome involves a disproportionately greater loss of motor power in the upper limbs compared to the lower limbs with varying degrees of sensory loss. It is usually seen after a hyper-extension injury of the cervical spine in a patient with pre-existing cervical canal stenosis, commonly secondary to osteoarthritis. The syndrome is thought to arise as a result of vascular compromise of the cord in the distribution of the anterior spinal artery. Brown–Sequard syndrome involves ipsilateral motor and proprioceptive loss and contralateral pain and temperature loss. Anterior cord syndrome is characterised by severe injury to most of the cord, with dorsal column sparing (preservation of proprioception and deep pressure sensation). Conus lesions involve damage to the sacral cord/lumbar nerve roots and produce reflex bowel and bladder function.

Trauma/orthopaedic surgery

115 COMPLICATIONS OF FRACTURES

1 E – Compartment syndrome

This is the typical description of compartment syndrome. This term refers to increased soft tissue pressure within an enclosed soft tissue compartment usually of the extremities (although it is possible to see abdominal compartment syndrome). Untreated it can lead to devastating muscle necrosis, contracture, nerve damage and ultimately severe functional impairment. Common causes of compartment syndrome include fractures (commonly tibial), soft tissue crush injuries, burns, gunshot wounds, surgery and vascular impairment. Clinical presentation, in a conscious patient, is severe pain, particularly on passive stretching of the muscle group involved. As time progresses paraesthesia, pallor, pulselessness and paralysis all begin to develop (the latter three at a stage where irreversible damage may already have occurred). Clinical suspicion with a relevant history should be enough to warrant surgical exploration and decompression via fasciotomy.

2 M – Myositis ossificans

This is a process whereby extraskeletal ossification occurs in muscle and soft tissue. Usually it arises after injury: commonly elbow fractures, elbow dislocations and injuries leading to large haematoma formation (eg soft tissue injuries of the thigh). It is thought to be related to joint mobilisation that is too early after injury, or too rigorous. Symptoms are as those described in the clinical scenario and treatment is rest, usually with immobilisation of the affected joint in a cast for a few weeks. In this way the accumulated calcification gradually reduces, and movement increases. Late excision may ultimately be required for non-resolution.

3 D – Avascular necrosis (AVN)

Bone death (osteonecrosis) is usually the result of impaired blood supply. This can occur by two mechanisms: interruption of arterial inflow (eg after a fracture), or obstruction of venous outflow (eg by lesions that infiltrate and block the venous sinusoids). In this case a fracture to the scaphoid has disrupted the local blood supply. Other common sites that have a propensity to become ischaemic, and hence develop AVN, include the femoral head and the body of the talus. On X-ray the distinctive feature of AVN is increased bone density (as a result of new bone ingrowth in the necrotic segment with disuse osteoporosis in the surrounding regions).

4 C – Associated injury: visceral

Fractures around the trunk can often be complicated by injuries to the underlying viscera. In this scenario blunt trauma to the chest with resultant rib fractures have led to a pneumothorax.

116 COMMON FRACTURE EPONYMS

1 K – Rolando's fracture

This description could be one of a Bennett's fracture, but the comminuted nature distinguishes it as a Rolando's fracture. There are usually three fragments forming either a Y-shape or a T-shape on radiograph.

2 N – Weber B fracture

The Weber (or Danis–Weber) classification describes the severity of tibiofibular ligament injury by the level of fibular fracture. This is a Weber B fracture as it is sited at the level of the syndesmosis. A Weber A fracture is infra-syndesmotic while a Weber C fracture occurs above the level of the syndesmosis. The Lauge–Hansen classification is an alternative method of describing fractures of the distal tibia and fibular. It takes into account foot position and direction of deforming forces, and is preferred by senior orthopaedic surgeons. For your purposes the Weber system is sufficient as the Lauge–Hansen is complex and not all fractures fit the classical pattern.

3 F – Garden III fracture

The Garden classification is used to describe intra-capsular fractures of the neck of the femur. It is important to distinguish these from extra-capsular fractures, as there is a bearing on blood supply, and ultimately, treatment. The capsule contributes the majority of the blood supply to the head of the femur, via the medial and lateral circumflex arteries from the profunda femoris. A compromise in the blood supply can result in avascular necrosis. The Garden system consists of four grades (I–IV) as follows:

- Garden I – incomplete or impacted fracture
- Garden II – non-displaced fracture through both cortices
- Garden III – minimally displaced fracture with rotation of the femoral head in the acetabulum
- Garden IV – completely displaced fracture of the head of femur (no continuity between the proximal and distal fragments).

4 A – Barton's fracture

This injury results from a fall onto an outstretched hand. The Barton fracture can be sub-divided into volar and dorsal types. It can be distinguished radiographically from Colles' or Smith's fractures by the presence of a dislocation or subluxation. This involves the rim of the distal radius, which can be dorsally or volarly displaced with the hand and carpus. The majority of these fractures require surgical reduction and fixation.

117 TREATMENT OPTIONS IN FRACTURE MANAGEMENT

1 A – Broad arm sling

Fractures of the clavicle, despite representing 5% of all fractures (and 44% of shoulder girdle fractures), seldom excite much interest. They are usually treated conservatively in a broad arm sling (or polysling), although surgical fixation may be indicated. Operative treatment is reserved for those patients with: open fractures, polytrauma, neurovascular injury (NB proximity of brachial plexus), compromise of the overlying skin, floating shoulder, symptomatic non-union and fractures of the lateral third proximal to, or between, the conoid and trapezoid ligaments.

2 D – Dynamic screw fixation

For an extracapsular fracture, where blood supply to the femoral head is not significantly compromised (such as that described in this scenario), the ideal method of fixation is with dynamic screw fixation, specifically a dynamic hip screw. This is a plate and sliding screw fixator that permits compression at the fracture site. It allows good anatomical fixation of the fracture and early mobilisation of the patient.

3 N – Traction

Paediatric femoral shaft fractures are commonly treated by skin or skeletal traction. This allows fracture union before the child then commences mobilisation in an appropriate cast. It is important to note that fixation of fractures in young children can disturb bone growth (particularly intramedullary nailing through an epiphyseal growth plate), leading to shortening and malformation of the affected limb. Hence it is restricted to the management of the polytraumatised child when plate fixation or external fixation may be used with care.

4 E – External fixation

Indications for external fixation in trauma encompass: compound (open) long bone fractures with extensive tissue devitalisation (especially of the tibia), closed fractures with degloving skin injuries, 'open book' pelvic fractures, polytrauma, peri-articular and metaphyseal fractures. The unique characteristics of external fixation include: rapid skeletal stabilisation using connecting frames and percutaneous pins, remote from the site of injury; versatility (different injuries with differing anatomy); ability to adjust alignment and fixation during fracture healing; and ease of access to surrounding soft tissues.

118 COMMON DISORDERS OF THE HAND

1 N – Trigger finger

This condition is caused by thickening of the flexor tendon, paratenon, or a narrowing of the flexor sheath. Consequently, the affected finger becomes locked in full flexion and will only extend after excessive voluntary effort, or assistance from the other hand. When extension begins it does so suddenly, and with a click, hence the name of the condition. The condition is usually painless. Steroid infiltration may be effective in mild cases, although surgical release of the proximal portion of the A1 pulley may be necessary.

2 J – Phalangeal endochondroma

This benign tumour is composed of mature, hyaline cartilage, and presents as a slow-growing mass within a phalanx. Pain, swelling or deformity of the affected finger may be evident. The presentation may be acute, with a 'pathological' fracture through the weakened cortex, as in the case described. There is a characteristic appearance on radiography. The usual opacity of the bony phalanx is lost, and the cavity of the mass appears radiolucent with stippled calcification. The cortex of the bone may be thinned as the internal mass expands. Treatment involves curettage followed by cancellous bone grafting.

3 K – Pulp space infection

Pulp space infections usually arise from minor penetrating injuries. Pressure in the infected compartment causes marked pain. Infection may spread into adjacent compartments because of infarction of surrounding tissues secondary to rapidly increasing pressure. Occasionally, this may lead to rupture through the overlying skin, or into the distal phalanx. Treatment should involve early incision and drainage, to avoid permanent loss of pulp tissue, and subsequent reduction of cushioning of the distal phalanx.

119 MONO AND POLYARTHRITIS

1 I – Septic arthritis

Joints can become infected by direct extension from a wound, by direct introduction (joint injection/arthroscopy), or by spread from acute osteomyelitis or haematogenously. Staphylococci and *Haemophilus influenzae* predominate, although other Gram-positive cocci and Gram-negative bacilli may be implicated. The infection usually starts in the synovial membrane, and a seropurulent exudate develops in the synovial fluid. There is progressive destruction of the articular cartilage, and vascular damage may lead to death of epiphyseal bone; hence the need for urgent diagnosis and appropriate treatment. The classic clinical feature is reluctance to move the joint, but swelling and erythema are commonly present. The joint is the maximal site of tenderness (differentiating it from acute osteomyelitis), and all joint movements are restricted. White cell count and erythrocyte sedimentation rate/C-reactive protein are invariably raised. Radiography is often unremarkable in the early stages. Treatment involves analgesia, appropriate antibiotics, joint aspiration, or occasionally formal open drainage.

2 E – Pseudogout

This condition involves acute or chronic arthritis secondary to deposition of calcium pyrophosphate or basic calcium phosphates. Pyrophosphate is generated in cartilage by enzyme activity, and combines with calcium ions to form crystals. In many cases it is idiopathic, although it may occur in hyperparathyroidism, hypothyroidism, acromegaly, or haemochromatosis. The clinical presentation is less severe and usually more chronic than with gout (urate crystal arthropathy in patients with hyperuricaemia). The fibrocartilage of the knee, pubic symphysis and intervertebral discs are most commonly affected, particularly in women over the age of 60 years. Radiography reveals calcification that usually appears as a line across the joint, but the synovial capsule and surrounding tendons may be calcified. The diagnosis is confirmed by demonstrating weakly positive bi-refringent rhomboid crystals in plane-polarised light.

3 K – Still's disease

Juvenile chronic arthritis (Still's disease) affects 1 in 1000 children, with 70% of those affected being female. At least two of joint pain, swelling, or limitation of movement, need to affect more than four joints for at least 3 months for the diagnosis to be accepted. Associated systemic symptoms of fever, macular rash and lymphadenopathy may predominate. Recurrent abdominal pain may occur secondary to bouts of mesenteric adenitis, as in the case presented. Hepatosplenomegaly, myocarditis and uveitis may complicate this condition. In 90% of cases the condition is seronegative and can only be confirmed by synovial biopsy. Chronic disease may lead to joint destruction, fibrosis and ankylosis, resulting in deformity. In addition, end-organ failure may supervene. It is differentiated from Reiter's syndrome (polyarthritis, urethritis, conjunctivitis) on account of no urethral involvement.

120 COMPLICATIONS OF RHEUMATOID ARTHRITIS

1 B – Boutonnière deformity

This scenario describes the typical changes that occur with a Boutonnière deformity. These transformations occur as a result of rupture of the middle slip of the extensor tendon. At this stage there is no more than a failure to extend the proximal interphalangeal joint; however, if the tendon is not repaired the lateral slips slide down towards the volar surface allowing the knuckle to 'buttonhole' through the extensor hood, causing the distal interphalangeal joint to be drawn into hyperextension.

2 E – Felty's syndrome

This haematological complication of rheumatoid arthritis was named after its pioneer: Augustus Felty (1934). The syndrome comprises seropositive (often high titres of rheumatoid factor) rheumatoid arthritis (frequently with relatively inactive synovitis), splenomegaly and neutropenia. It usually occurs in longstanding disease, and recurrent, severe infections are a common complication, as is vasculitis (leg ulcers and mononeuritis), lymphadenopathy and pigmentation. Resultant hypersplenism (see question 56) may require splenectomy.

3 K – Pleural effusion

Typically, pleural effusion is unilateral and arises in seropositive men over the age of 45 years. It often precedes articular manifestations (arthritis), and unlike most other extra-articular complications, can occur early on in the disease. The effusion can be chronic and associated with significant pleural thickening. Other pulmonary manifestations include: rheumatoid nodules (less than 1% of cases) which can cavitate and need to be differentiated from primary and metastatic malignancy; and bronchiolitis obliterans, an illness characterised by rapid onset of breathlessness, progressing over a few months to complete incapacity or death. Pulmonary function tests show considerable reduction in vital capacity, with gross hyperinflation, although the chest X-ray is virtually normal. Interstitial disease occurs in 1–5% of patients and generally progresses slowly, but may remain stable or even regress over the years.

4 D – Carpal tunnel syndrome

Carpal tunnel syndrome is a nerve compression syndrome that is frequently associated with rheumatoid arthritis. Swelling, inflammation and tenosynovitis of the anterior tendons as they pass under the flexor retinaculum cause compression of the median nerve with resultant tingling and pain in its region of distribution. Chronic pressure leads to wasting of the muscles supplied by the median nerve at this level (**LOAF** – ie **L**umbricals (first two), **O**pponens pollicis, **A**bductor pollicis brevis and **F**lexor pollicis brevis). The causes should also be memorised.

121 UPPER LIMB INJURIES

1 L – Posterior dislocation of the shoulder

This frequently missed injury should be suspected following a seizure or electric shock. The mechanism involves either a direct blow to the front of the shoulder or forced internal rotation when the arm is abducted. Clinical features are as described. In addition, the anterior contour of the shoulder may be flattened with prominence of the coracoid. Anteroposterior radiographs may look virtually normal, but the medially rotated humeral head appears globe-shaped (light bulb sign). Treatment involves closed reduction, which is maintained by a shoulder spica.

2 J – Fractured shaft of humerus

This injury occurs at all ages but is most common in elderly osteoporotic individuals. The extensive bruising is characteristic. The diagnosis is supported in this case by the finding of a wrist drop, which has been caused by a radial nerve injury where it lies in the spiral groove of the humerus. Treatment is with a hanging cast, the weight of which maintains reduction. In closed injuries the nerve is seldom divided and the wrist may be splinted while the injury recovers. Fractures to the humeral shaft may be pathological and any occurring following minor trauma should be viewed with suspicion.

3 K – Olecranon fracture

Two types of injury are commonly seen. The first is a comminuted fracture following direct trauma to the point of the elbow. The second is a traction injury to the olecranon resulting in a transverse fracture. This typically occurs following a fall onto the hand with the triceps muscle contracted. Transverse fractures tend to cause disruption to the extensor mechanism of the elbow as in the case described. Displaced fractures may result in a palpable gap. Treatment of non-displaced fractures involves immobilisation in a cast followed by supervised mobilisation. Displaced fractures are treated by open reduction and internal fixation. Methods available include tension band wiring and plating.

122 BACK PAIN

1 F – Osteomyelitis

In approximately half of cases of osteomyelitis of the spine there is a history of recent pelvic surgery, urinary tract infection, cutaneous sepsis, or diabetes mellitus. It is likely that haematogenous spread occurs via the vertebral venous plexus (Batson's plexus) to the spine. The most common infecting organism is *Staphylococcus aureus,* although Gram-negative organisms occur in association with urinary tract infection. The pain is usually worse in the recumbent position, and the patient is frequently pyrexial. White cell count, erythrocyte sedimentation rate and C-reactive protein are raised. Blood cultures, computed tomography, radioisotope or magnetic resonance scanning may all be helpful in making the diagnosis. Treatment is with rest, analgesia and appropriate antibiotics. Occasionally, surgery is required to 'decompress' the spine.

2 C – Metastatic carcinoma

This case describes the disseminated presentation of carcinoma of the bronchus with secondary involvement of the lumbar spine. The majority of extradural spinal tumours are metastatic. The most common primary sites include the breast, bronchus, prostate, kidney, thyroid gland, or haemopoietic malignancies. The pain is non-mechanical (unrelated to physical activity), and is aggravated by recumbency. Occasionally, vertebral collapse may lead to presentation with profound neurological deficit. Plain radiographs may be normal early in the disease, and so isotope and magnetic resonance imaging may be more useful. Metastatic disease without clinical or radiological evidence of neurological compression is treated with radiotherapy, chemotherapy, or hormone manipulation. Occasionally, anterior or posterior decompression surgery +/− fixation is required.

3 E – Osteoporosis

This condition is defined by the World Health Organisation as 'a progressive systemic skeletal disease characterised by low bone mass and microarchitectural deterioration of bone tissue with increased bone fragility and susceptibility to fracture'. Osteoporosis results in 200, 000 fractures per year (one-third of all women sustain one or more osteoporotic fractures), and leads to significant pain and individual disability. Bone density decreases with increasing age, immobility and postmenopausally in women. Conditions leading to secondary osteoporosis include: thyroid dysfunction, Cushing's syndrome, premature (< 51 years)/iatrogenic (total abdominal hysterectomy with bilateral salpingo-oophorectomy) menopause, rheumatoid arthritis, drugs (corticosteroids, alcohol, anticonvulsants). Measurement of bone mineral density can be performed using dual energy X-ray absorptiometry scanning, and the hip is the site with the highest predictive value. Hormone replacement therapy, and bisphosphonates (etidronate/alendronate) prevent bone loss and decrease the risk of fractures; vitamin D and calcium supplements decrease the risk of hip and other fractures in the frail elderly.

123 BONE AND SOFT TISSUE TUMOURS

Primary tumours of bone and soft tissue are uncommon. They usually present with unremitting pain, swelling and loss of function. They may also present with a pathological fracture, a joint effusion or systemic symptoms when there is metastatic spread. In the diagnosis of bone tumours, the frequency of various tumours, the patient's age, the bone affected and the location of the lesion within the bone, and its radiological appearances are all important.

1 N – Osteosarcoma (osteogenic sarcoma)

This is one of the commonest primary malignant bone tumours affecting the young with a slight male predominance. There is also a second peak in incidence in the elderly related to Paget's disease. The long bone metaphyses are usually affected, most commonly around the knee. Blood-borne metastases develop early and spread to the lungs and other parts of the skeleton. Cortical penetration with peri-osteal elevation gives rise to 'Codman's triangle' on X-ray. In addition, a characteristic sunray appearance may be evident on a plain radiograph as a result of new bone formation. In terms of histology, some may be largely fibroblastic, others are osteoblastic (with pleomorphic cells), some comprise chondroid osteoblasts, and they may even be highly vascular (telangiectatic). All form osteoid and/or bone-incorporating malignant cells. Computed tomography and magnetic resonance scanning are important in staging. Treatment involves chemotherapy combined with wide surgical excision (with limb salvage if possible). Five-year survival rates of 60% can be expected in those without distant metastases.

2 C – Chondrosarcoma

This is a malignant tumour of cartilage that affects the flat bones, vertebrae, girdles and the proximal limb bones in middle-aged patients. X-ray images may be diagnostic and reveal localised bone destruction, punctuated by mottled densities from calcification or ossification, as in the case described. Histological differentiation from enchondroma and osteosarcoma may be difficult. Treatment is similar to that for osteosarcomas, and 5-year survival rates are approximately 50%.

3 D – Ewing's sarcoma

This aggressive tumour is unusual in that it often affects the mid-diaphysis (shaft) of the bone, typically in children and adolescents. It is slightly less prevalent than osteosarcoma. It may masquerade as an osteomyelitis. Metastases arise in the liver, lung and other bones. Radiography reveals a characteristic 'onion-skin' appearance of the periosteum. Survival rates of 60% can be achieved at 5 years with the use of combined surgery, radiotherapy and chemotherapy.

124 PAINFUL CONDITIONS OF THE FOOT

1 H – Morton's metatarsalgia

The description is a classical presentation of this condition. The exact aetiology is unclear; it is thought to occur following entrapment of a digital nerve between the metatarsal heads with secondary thickening and formation of a neuroma. The nerve most commonly affected lies between the third and fourth metatarsal heads. Pain is usually acute and may be associated with a sensory disturbance in the distribution of the nerve. If symptoms are troublesome treatment is by excision of the neuroma.

2 G – March fracture

This is a metatarsal stress fracture, usually of the second or third metatarsal, which occurs in young adults after a period of unaccustomed walking. The initial complaint is that of pain in the forefoot and the affected bone feels thick and tender. The fracture may not be evident on initial X-rays of the foot but eventually reveals itself by the appearance of abundant callus. The condition is self limiting with no long-term sequelae. Treatment is symptomatic.

3 C – Gout

This condition is the commonest form of inflammatory joint disease in men over 40 with the first metatarsophalangeal joint affected in over 90% of cases. The condition closely resembles septic arthritis; however, there is an absence of systemic features of infection. The primary cause is hyperuricaemia and there may be a precipitating cause such as alcohol excess or foods high in purines and diuretics. Treatment during the acute phase is with anti-inflammatory drugs followed by a xanthine oxidase inhibitor, eg allopurinol to prevent further episodes.

4 F – Hammer toe

The clinical findings are characteristic with pain occurring as a result of callosities forming over the pressure areas. This should not be confused with claw toes where there is hyperextension of the metatarsophalangeal joint and flexion of both the interphalangeal joints. If pain is severe, treatment is by excision arthrodesis.

5 K – Sever's disease

This condition is the most likely cause of a painful heel in a child and is a form of osteochondritis of the calcaneal epithesis. Pain and tenderness occur close to the insertion of the Achilles tendon. Radiographs may demonstrate epiphyseal fragmentation or sclerosis. The condition is self limiting with symptoms controlled by means of a pressure-relieving pad.

125 THE PAINFUL KNEE

1 L – Rheumatoid arthritis

This can occasionally start in the knee as a monoarticular synovitis. With chronicity, the joint may become increasingly deformed. Although deformity can also occur (with chronic pain and swelling) in osteoarthritis, a valgus deformity is characteristic of rheumatoid arthritis whereas a varus deformity is frequently seen with severe osteoarthritis.

2 B – Chondromalacia patellae

Softening of the articular cartilage of the patella is often associated with anterior knee pain in teenage girls. The exact aetiology is unknown, however, it is thought to result from overload of the patellar articular surface as a result of mal-tracking of the patella during flexion and extension. On clinical examination, pain can be elicited by the patella friction test. Treatment is rest, analgesia and physiotherapy.

3 I – Osteochondritis dessicans

This is a condition where a small osteocartilaginous fragment separates from one of the femoral condyles (usually the medial condyle) and is rendered avascular. Patients tend to be young and present with intermittent pain and swelling of the knee. Attacks of 'locking' may occur as the loose body becomes trapped between the joint surfaces. Between attacks the loose body may be palpable, particularly in the suprapatellar pouch. Treatment involves removal of the loose body if small. Large fragments may be fixed back into position, particularly if complete separation has not occurred.

126 KNEE INJURIES

1 F – Meniscal tear

Meniscal tears in the young adult typically result from a rotational stress upon the flexed weight-bearing knee joint. This mechanism of injury is often the same for anterior cruciate ligament (ACL) rupture (and frequently these injuries co-exist). The clues in this clinical scenario that point to meniscal damage, over ACL rupture, include: the symptom of locking (true locking is the inability to fully straighten the knee), which indicates a mechanical blockage within the knee; and the delayed onset of swelling (characteristically > 6 h after injury). The swelling is an effusion as a result of the synovial reaction, in contrast to the haemarthrosis seen in ACL rupture, which is an immediate phenomenon. Symptomatic meniscal tears warrant arthroscopic intervention.

2 B – Extensor mechanism disruption

Any part of the extensor mechanism can be damaged at any age; however, there are common patterns of injury. In the middle-aged and elderly the quadriceps tendon and muscle tend to be compromised more readily. Patellar fractures are seen more often in the young and middle-aged, with tibial tuberosity avulsion occurring in younger age ranges. Patellar tendon rupture can happen at any age. In this scenario the man has ruptured his quadriceps tendon. This results from forced contraction of the extensor mechanism with the foot planted on the floor and can arise from a simple stumble or fall. Clinical examination may reveal a haemarthrosis and there is inevitably a palpable gap in the tendon at the site of rupture. The patient is unable to perform a straight leg raise (particularly against resistance) or to actively straighten the knee. Direct repair of the tendon using non-absorbable material is required, because without intervention the extensor mechanism is severely compromised and the patient is unable to walk properly.

3 A – Anterior cruciate ligament (ACL) injury

Injury to the ACL is fairly common. Patients often describe a non-contact, deceleration, twisting injury (although sometimes the mechanism is of hyperextension). In over 50% of cases the history will include hearing a 'pop' or feeling a sensation of something tearing inside the knee, with early-onset swelling. (NB Up to 80% of patients attending Casualty with an acute haemarthrosis, have sustained an injury to their ACL and of these, 60% will have another associated pathology within the knee.) Specific examination of the ACL via the anterior draw and Lachman tests should be undertaken. Routine use of magnetic resonance imaging is probably unnecessary;

however, it does have the advantage of delineating other associated ligamentous, meniscal, or bony damage. With regard to long-term management of ACL injuries there is still debate as to the necessity and timing of reconstructive surgery.

4 K – Proximal tibio-fibular dislocation

This is an uncommon injury and tends to be caused by twisting of the weight-bearing flexed knee. It can occur as an isolated injury or in association with major trauma. Classically known as 'horseback rider's knee', it is more commonly associated with parachute jumping (requiring a considerable amount of force). Hypermobile individuals (eg those with Ehlers–Danlos syndrome) are more susceptible. Examination reveals tenderness over the proximal tibio-fibular joint and movement of the ankle tends to cause pain in the knee. It is paramount to assess the integrity of the common peroneal nerve, as it passes close to the joint and can easily be injured. Reduction is effected by pressure over the fibular head with the knee flexed.

127 THE CHILDHOOD LIMP

1 G – Slipped upper femoral epiphysis

This condition occurs during the pubertal growth spurt and the description of the patient is typical; an overweight boy, aged 13–15 who is sexually underdeveloped. The condition also occurs less commonly in unusually tall and thin children. The onset of pain may be either acute, chronic, or acute on chronic. Examination findings are as described. Treatment is by internal fixation of the slipped epiphysis with or without a corrective osteotomy.

2 E – Perthes' disease

The condition tends to occur between the ages of 4 and 7 when the blood supply is dependent on the lateral epiphyseal vessels, which run in the retinaculum. Trauma to the joint with a secondary effusion may compromise these vessels with consequent necrosis of the femoral head. Initial presentation is with symptoms and signs of an irritable hip; pain in the affected joint and a reduced range of movement. With time the pain subsides and movement returns; however, abduction and internal rotation remain limited. Changes may only become apparent on X-ray after several years and as such these patients need to be followed up carefully. Treatment is directed at 'containment', with the aim of ensuring the femoral head remains in the acetabulum by preventing lateral displacement of the femoral head. This is usually achieved by the use of an abduction splint.

3 D – Non-specific transient tenosynovitis

This is the commonest cause of a limp with hip pain in a child and is self limiting in its natural history. Onset of pain tends to be sudden and of variable intensity. Examination findings are as described, and initial investigations tend to be normal. The condition tends to resolve after a few days of bed rest with analgesia and gentle traction applied to the affected limb.

4 H – Still's disease

The history is characteristic with an episodic fever associated with arthritis. Despite the presentation with a fever there are no other features to suggest a septic arthritis; pyogenic arthritis tends to occur at a younger age (usually less than 2), the child appears unwell and the affected joint is hot, swollen and held absolutely still. Rheumatoid factor is negative and antinuclear antibodies may be present. The erythrocyte sedimentation rate tends to be raised. Three types have been described, systemic, pauciarticular and polyarticular. Initial treatment is with non-steroidal anti-inflammatory drugs.

Urology

128 HAEMATURIA

Haematuria may occur as a result of renal, ureteric, bladder, prostatic and urethral causes. The following pathological processes are usually implicated: trauma, infection, tumours, or stones. In addition, bleeding diatheses may manifest as haematuria. When investigations fail to identify a cause, medical disorders of the kidney should be sought by a nephrologist.

1 H – Polycystic kidney disease

Adult polycystic kidney disease is an autosomal dominant condition (the *PKD* gene is on chromosome 6) that affects 1 in 1000 of the population, and accounts for approximately 10% of cases of chronic renal failure. Polycystic changes are always bilateral and present from early childhood to old-age. Patients most commonly present with bilateral loin pain, haematuria, hypertension, proteinuria, progressive renal failure and bilateral abdominal masses. Cysts arise anywhere along the nephron, may reach 3–4 cm in diameter, and so compress the surrounding parenchyma. Forty per cent of patients have associated liver cysts, and 10–30% have berry aneurysms. Intravenous urogram, ultrasound scan and computed tomography are helpful. Management is aimed at controlling hypertension, treating infections, and monitoring for renal failure. Surgery is only indicated for bleeding or intractable pain.

2 L – Renal papillary necrosis

Renal papillary necrosis affects the distal portion of the renal pyramid. It is seen in association with analgesic abuse and diabetes mellitus, which provide clues in distinguishing it clinically from urolithiasis. The condition is caused by infarction of renal pyramids as a result of co-existing arteriosclerosis or an acute vasculitis. Clinical presentation may be related to symptoms of urinary tract infection, such as recurrent fever, malaise, dysuria, flank pain, proteinuria, haematuria and leukocytosis. Passage of sloughed papillae can cause renal colic, ureteric obstruction and, rarely, urinoma. Rarely, renal papillary necrosis can present as acute oliguric renal failure. In the advanced stage, renal function may be impaired and anaemia and uraemia may be noted. The patient may witness the passage of 'tissue' (sloughed papillae), rather than 'grit' (calculi) in the urine, as in the case described. Early in the disease, renal size and function are preserved. Function may deteriorate with eventual renal failure in the later stages of the disease. Radiography may demonstrate a wavy renal outline with tracks of contrast, ring shadows as a result of sloughing of papillae, and an egg-in-a-cup appearance characteristic of renal papillary necrosis.

3 N – Urethral caruncle

A urethral caruncle is an inflammatory tumour, 1–1.5 cm in diameter, of the urethral meatus in women, most frequently in the 6 o'clock position. They are very vascular and covered with transitional epithelium. Although frequently asymptomatic, they may give rise to spotting and microscopic haematuria. Oestrogen deficiency is implicated in the aetiology. The diagnosis is clinical, although failure to respond to oestrogen therapy should prompt excisional biopsy to exclude a more sinister pathology.

129 INVESTIGATION OF URINARY TRACT DISORDERS

1 I – Magnetic resonance imaging (MRI)
The standard primary investigation for haematuria and loin pain (with or without a mass) is an ultrasound, which has already been undertaken for this patient. If a renal cyst demonstrates a solid intracystic element or an irregular or calcified wall, as in this case, it is regarded as potentially malignant and requires further imaging for staging. This is usually completed by computed tomography (CT) scanning of the chest and abdomen, with intravenous contrast administration. In patients who have a prior history of reaction to contrast, MRI is the chosen modality for staging assessment. In the staging of patients with renal carcinoma MRI appears more accurate in delineating inferior vena cava or renal vein involvement, compared with CT.

2 C – Computed tomography urography (CTU)
Although this woman has a nephrostomy tube sited and this could be used for antegrade contrast studies of her urinary tract, she has raised urea and creatinine that could be exacerbated by contrast use. CTU has the advantage in this scenario of allowing rapid visualisation of the renal tract without the need for contrast injection. It has a high sensitivity for ureteric stones. If no renal tract stone is identified, CTU has the advantage over intravenous urogram, and retrograde or antegrade ureteropyelography, in that it can demonstrate other intra-abdominal pathologies that might be causing upper tract obstruction.

3 F – Intravenous ureterogram (IVU)
The gold standard first investigation (cystourethroscopy may often be required subsequently) for investigating painless macroscopic haematuria is still IVU. Although many urology departments may combine plain abdominal kidney, ureter and bladder X-ray with renal tract ultrasound it is important to recognise that ultrasonography is less sensitive than IVU for detecting tumours of the upper tract, which comprise 1–2% of all urothelial tumours.

130 BLADDER OUTFLOW OBSTRUCTION

1 O – Urethral stricture

This gentleman is likely to have developed a urethral stricture. Strictures can result from an inflammatory process or trauma. Historically, gonorrhoea was a common cause of stricture, but nowadays they tend to arise secondary to traumatic urethral instrumentation (eg long-term catheterisation, cystoscopy, or as a result of large-bore resectoscope use in transurethral resection of the prostate). Prolonged urethral catheterisation, such as in this case, can lead to stricture. This is particularly true in this scenario when, following coronary bypass grafting, urethral ischaemia in a patient with cardiovascular disease may be an exacerbating factor.

2 A – Benign prostatic hypertrophy (BPH)

The presenting symptoms and prostate-specific antigen (PSA) result in this clinical picture point to a diagnosis of BPH. Lower urinary tract symptoms (LUTS) can vary between irritative storage symptoms (frequency, urgency, nocturia) and voiding symptoms (hesitancy, poor flow, intermittent flow and post-micturition dribbling). The PSA is within normal limits for age (age-specific value for 70+ can be up to 6.5 ng/ml), although in BPH, because of the increased prostatic volume, the level can be higher, making it more difficult to rule out prostatic cancer. Management can initially be via drug therapy (α-blockers or 5α-reductase inhibitors, eg Finasteride) but ultimately, if patients remain symptomatic, they will be offered a transurethral resection of the prostate (TURP).

3 F – Clot retention

The cause of this man's acute retention is clot within the bladder. His history of frank haematuria on a background of surgery for transitional cell cancer resection (following transurethral resection of bladder tumour) makes this the clear diagnosis. Immediate management will require the insertion of a rigid three-way irrigating catheter (a normal flexible Foley catheter is likely to obstruct with clot after a short period). This allows perfusion of the bladder with a normal saline irrigation fluid until the bleeding has settled. More persistent bleeding may require repeat rigid cystoscopy and diathermy to the affected area. Obviously a full set of bloods should be drawn and transfusion should be undertaken as necessary.

4 G – Detrusor-external sphincter dyssynergia (DESD)

The higher centre for co-ordination of bladder with urethral function lies within the pons and is known as the pontine micturition centre (PMC). The cell bodies of the parasympathetic motor fibres to the detrusor muscle

(S2–S4) and somatic motor fibres innervating the striated urethral sphincter (S2–S4) are located in the sacral spinal cord. They receive descending impulses from the PMC, which is therefore responsible for ensuring that co-ordinated contraction of the bladder and relaxation of the sphincter occur simultaneously, allowing normal voiding. In DESD the PMC is disconnected from the sacral spinal cord (classically by spinal cord injury) and patients lose the appropriate bladder–sphincter synchronisation. In a reversal of normal function, when their bladder contracts it does so forcibly against a closed urethral sphincter and hence these patients develop retention with very high bladder pressures leading to renal back pressure and renal failure (note raised urea and creatinine). As the patient tries to pass urine the voiding cystourethrogram shows the external sphincter (positioned between the prostatic and bulbar urethra) continuing to contract when it should be relaxing.

131 DISORDERS OF THE PROSTATE

1 B – Benign prostatic hyperplasia

Benign prostatic hyperplasia (BPH) is the commonest disease to affect middle-aged men. The aetiology remains unknown, although some form of androgen imbalance appears important. The gland is enlarged by nodules of variable size arising in the inner (peri-urethral) portion. Enlargement of the inner zone of the gland tends to produce atrophy of the outer gland, which forms a pseudocapsule to the prostate. Consequently, smooth enlargement of the gland is characteristic of BPH on digital examination. Microscopically, these nodules are composed of proliferating glands and fibromuscular stroma. The relative obstruction of urinary flow produces the classical 'obstructive' symptoms associated with BPH, namely, hesitancy, poor flow and terminal dribbling. Such symptoms are relatively successfully addressed by surgical 'decompression' (eg transurethral resection of the prostate). However, the bladder detrusor compensates for increased outflow resistance with muscular hypertrophy and an increase in collagen, resulting in trabeculation. Trabeculation is asymptomatic but the detrusor becomes increasingly irritable, giving rise to 'irritative' symptoms of urinary frequency, nocturia and urgency. Such symptoms are not usually addressed by surgery, and are best treated medically (eg anti-cholinergics). With progressive obstruction, chronic retention of urine secondary to incomplete bladder emptying may precipitate infections, and in the long-term may lead to chronic renal failure. Patients may experience acute retention of urine. Management includes α-blockers, 5α-reductase inhibitors and, in resistant, cases transurethral or transvesical resection of the prostate.

2 F – Prostatic abscess

Effective treatment of acute prostatitis with antibiotics has reduced the prevalence of prostatic abscesses. However, they may be seen in patients with immunocompromise. The clinical picture is of systemic sepsis as a result of abscess formation, and occasionally, outflow obstruction/retention of urine when the collection is large, as in the case described. The initial treatment is with parenteral antibiotics. Transurethral incision may be required to drain the abscess if medical treatment is ineffective.

3 C – Carcinoma of the prostate

Carcinoma of the prostate is usually an adenocarcinoma of acinar form. Its aetiology remains unknown. Most arise in the peripheral part of the gland, and so it is amenable to detection on rectal examination. Presentation may be asymptomatic (incidental finding), with a palpable nodule on per rectum examination, with LUTI's (usually obstructive in nature), although given the peripheral location of tumours there is usually considerable involvement of the gland by the time outflow obstruction develops. Patients may also present with disseminated metastatic disease (bone and/or perineal pain), or locally advanced disease, encircling the rectum and causing mechanical obstruction of the large intestine, as in the clinical scenario presented.

132 THEME: URINARY INCONTINENCE

For continence to exist, urethral pressure must exceed intravesical pressure at all times. Urinary incontinence is defined by the International Continence Society as 'the involuntary loss of urine which is objectively demonstrable and a social or hygienic problem'. It may be classified into urethral or extra-urethral conditions.

Urethral causes include
- *urethral sphincter incompetence*
- *detrusor overactivity (uninhibited detrusor contractions)*
- *overflow incontinence (eg secondary to retention of urine/faecal impaction/uterovaginal prolapse/drugs/urethral strictures/detrusor hypotonia etc)*
- *urinary tract infection*
- *urethral diverticulum*
- *functional (impaired cognition/intellectual function/immobility etc).*

Extra-urethral causes include
- *congenital abnormalities (eg ectopic ureter/bladder exstrophy)*
- *fistula formation (ureteric/vesical/vagina).*

1 I – Urethral sphincter incompetence

This has recently, and more accurately, been re-defined as 'urodynamic stress incontinence'. Consequently, it is a 'urodynamic diagnosis'. It is defined as the involuntary loss of urine when intravesical pressure exceeds the maximum urethral closure pressure in the absence of detrusor overactivity. It occurs as a result of incompetence of the urethral sphincter (hence its former name), which can be the result of weakness in any component of the sphincter mechanism (supporting structures, eg pubo-urethral and vesical ligaments), intrinsic sphincter mechanism, or extrinsic sphincter mechanism (puborectalis). It is more common in women, because of their anatomically shorter and straighter urethra. Presentation is commonly with incontinence provoked by 'stresses' that increase intra-abdominal pressure (eg coughing, sneezing, abdominal masses etc). In the first instance, treatment may be conservative [physiotherapy/mechanical devices/pharmacological agents (oestrogens)] or surgical (suspension/sling procedures/peri-urethral bulking agents).

2 C – Detrusor overactivity

Detrusor overactivity (DO) refers to objective contraction (spontaneous or on provocation) during the filling phase of cystometry, while the patient is attempting to inhibit micturition. It is, therefore, a urodynamic (cystometrographic) diagnosis. The contractions precipitate urinary urgency, and may result in leakage of urine ('urge incontinence'). The pathophysiology of DO remains poorly understood, and so it is termed idiopathic in the majority of cases. However, it may occur secondary to neuropathic lesions (multiple sclerosis/spinal injury/cerebrovascular accidents/Parkinsonism) or bladder outflow obstruction in men, as in the scenario presented. In the case of chronic obstruction, there is associated trabeculation (muscular hypertrophy and an increase in collagen) and increasing bladder irritability. Management of DO involves behavioural therapy (bladder drill), pharmacological manipulation (anti-cholinergic agents/calcium-channel blockers/anti-diuretics/hormone replacement therapy), and in severe refractory cases augmentation cystoplasty or more rarely urinary diversion.

3 F – Fistulation

A history of constant, uncontrollable loss of urine in an otherwise mentally intact individual should alert you to the presence of a fistula. Vesicovaginal, and less commonly urethrovaginal, fistulae usually occur secondary to gynaecological surgery in the developed world. By contrast, obstetric injury is the most common aetiology in the developing world. Assessment of such patients is clinical (examination under anaesthesia with dye insertion) and radiological (micturating cystogram). Repair is surgical.

133 SCROTAL SWELLINGS

1 M – Varicocoele

This is a condition of varicosities of the pampiniform plexus of veins (ie varicose veins of the spermatic cord) and is present in 15–25% of all men. They usually manifest first in adolescence and are more common on the left. This is explained by the venous drainage of the left testicular vein into the left renal vein at right angles (the right testicular vein drains obliquely into the inferior vena cava). Absent or incompetent valves at this junction with the left renal vein lead to back pressure, and the formation of the varicocoele. On examination with the patient standing the varicocoele is said to feel like a 'bag of worms'; it cannot be felt supine as the veins are empty. Usually varicocoeles are managed conservatively (close-fitting underwear, reassurance, analgesia for testicular ache); however, troublesome varicosities can be treated by radiological embolisation, or by surgical ligation of the testicular veins in the inguinal canal.

2 K – Testicular torsion

The classical age, history and clinical presentation in this scenario clearly points to testicular torsion. The commonest age for torsion is between 10 and 15 years and the problem is very uncommon over the age of 25 years. The majority of torsions occur spontaneously, often in the early hours of the morning; however, some follow minor trauma (eg blow to the scrotum during sport or while mounting a bicycle). In young sexually active men it may be difficult to distinguish between an acute epididymo-orchitis and testicular torsion. Surgical exploration is compulsory.

3 D – Epididymal cyst

Epididymal cysts are fluid-filled swellings connected to the epididymis and are thought to be derived from the collecting tubules of the epididymis. Most occur in men over the age of 40 years who complain of a slowly enlarging, non-tender bulge in the scrotum. Clinically they are as described in the scenario above. The differential diagnosis is that of a hydrocoele, but the epididymal cyst can easily be distinguished because of its position above and behind the superior pole of the testis. The fluid of a hydrocoele surrounds the testis and usually makes the testis impalpable.

4 F – Orchitis

This man's history of fever, malaise and parotitis indicates infection with the mumps virus (a systemic paramyxovirus). Orchitis occurs in up to 20% of post-pubertal men that contract the virus, commencing 4–6 days after the onset of the parotid gland swelling and lasting 7–10 days. Diagnosis is confirmed by the rising titre of anti-mumps antibody. Treatment is supportive (bed rest, analgesia and scrotal support). Mumps orchitis can be complicated by testicular atrophy. If the orchitis is bilateral fertility may be impaired.

134 HEMISCROTAL PAIN

1 L – Torsion of testicular appendage

There are four testicular appendages, which represent embryological remnants. These are the appendix testis (hydatid of Morgagni); the para-epididymis (organ of Giraldes); vasa aberrantia; and the appendix epididymis (pedunculated hydatid). The appendix testis undergoes torsion in 90% of cases. Torsion of an appendage is more common in boys under the age of 11 years than torsion of the testis. Similarly, acute epididymo-orchitis is unusual in young boys, unless there is an anatomical abnormality. The onset of pain is acute, and there is usually oedema of the cord. There may be an associated hydrocoele, making palpation of the twisted appendage difficult. Treatment involves exploration (also allowing absolute exclusion of testicular torsion) and removal of the appendage.

2 C – Fournier's gangrene

This is necrotising subcutaneous infection of the scrotum. The initial description by Fournier was in young healthy men, without obvious cause. Nowadays, the condition is most commonly seen in middle-aged or elderly gentlemen; there are frequently contributory factors such as local perineal/peri-anal or lower urinary tract surgery and immunocompromise (eg diabetes mellitus). Streptococci and *Clostridium perfringens* are usually implicated, and infection results in vascular thrombosis, subcutaneous tissue necrosis and eventually gangrene. The infection follows the same path as extravasation of urine, spreading into the perineum and lower abdominal wall. Treatment involves aggressive broad-spectrum antibiotic therapy, and emergency wide surgical excision of affected tissue.

3 A – Acute epididymo-orchitis

The aetiology of this infection varies with age. In young boys it is usually a bacterial infection associated with a structural abnormality of the lower genitourinary system. In young men it is most commonly sexually transmitted in origin, with *Chlamydia* and *Neisseria gonorrhoeae* commonly implicated. In older men it usually relates to prostatism, chronic retention of urine and/or instrumentation of the lower urinary tract. There is usually gradual onset of pain and swelling over several hours or days. There may be associated lower urinary tract symptoms. A swollen, tender epididymis may be palpable, but it may also fuse with the testis, forming a large inflammatory mass. A careful history and examination is crucial in establishing the correct diagnosis, and differentiating the problem from torsion. There may be associated bacteriuria. Treatment is with broad-spectrum antibiotics, with the addition of doxycycline (to cover *Chlamydia*) if an acquired cause is expected.

135 RENAL MASSES

1 A – Hydronephrosis

Hydronephrosis refers to dilatation of the renal pelvis and calyces associated with progressive atrophy of the kidney as a result of the obstruction of outflow of urine. Such obstruction may affect the upper urinary tract (ie ureteric obstruction), potentially resulting in unilateral hydronephrosis, or the lower urinary tract (bladder outflow obstruction etc), which usually results in bilateral hydronephrosis. Ureteric obstruction may be the result of congenital pelviureteric junction obstruction, or intraluminal (stones/tumours) or intramural (primary megaureter) pathology. It may occur secondary to extrinsic compression in the retroperitoneum (eg malignant disease/inflammatory disease/aneurysms/retroperitoneal fibrosis etc). Fibrosis around an aortic graft may result in ureteric obstruction, as in the case described. There may be associated impairment of renal function, particularly if the obstruction is bilateral. Ultrasound scanning will confirm that hydronephrosis is the cause of the renal enlargement. Treatment is directed towards the cause of the obstruction.

2 B – Nephroblastoma (Wilm's tumour)

This tumour is the commonest intra-abdominal malignancy in children under the age of 10 years. It is composed of primitive renal tubules, primitive renal blastoma-like mesenchyme, and fibroblast-like spindled cells. The peak incidence is between 2 and 4 years but cases may present during adolescence or even adulthood. The child is usually well, unlike in cases of neuroblastoma from which nephroblastoma **must** be distinguished. The commonest presentation is with an abdominal mass. Haematuria, pain, hypertension and intestinal obstruction may occur. Metastases occur to the liver. Treatment involves surgical excision and aggressive chemotherapy and radiotherapy. Five-year survival is in the order of 90%.

3 C – Peri-nephric abscess

Acute bacterial infections of the kidney form a spectrum ranging from relatively simple infection resulting in acute cystitis/pyelonephritis through to peri-nephric abscess formation. It is often difficult to clearly differentiate these on clinical grounds alone because they all present with localised symptoms of infection affecting the urinary tract, coupled with a degree of systemic effects (malaise, rigors, pyrexia, raised white count etc). Severe infection of the urinary tract may lead to pyonephrosis, particularly if the outflow of the kidney is obstructed by the presence of stones, as alluded to in the case scenario presented. Such a collection may discharge into the surrounding peri-renal tissue forming a peri-nephric abscess. Radiology is essential in differentiating between the various forms of acute infection. Treatment involves appropriate broad-spectrum antibiotics, and percutaneous or open drainage as required. An obstructed infected kidney is an indication for emergency nephrostomy.

136 TUMOURS OF THE GENITOURINARY TRACT

1 J – Transitional cell carcinoma of the bladder

Carcinoma of the bladder has a peak incidence in the seventh decade of life, and is three times more common in men. Many epidemiological studies have also shown a clear association with cigarette smoking. Ninety per cent of cancers are transitional cell carcinoma (TCC) in origin. Squamous cell carcinoma occurs frequently where bilharzial infections of the bladder are prevalent, and secondary to chronic infection with irritation (eg catheterised paraplegics/bladder stones). TCC demonstrate two patterns of growth: papillary and infiltrating. Haematuria is the cardinal symptom and may occur towards the end of micturition as a result of compression on the tumour as the bladder contracts to empty. Large tumours may give rise to irritative symptoms, and so such symptoms must not be assumed to be secondary to infection in older individuals, particularly if persistent or occurring in the absence of microbiological evidence of infection, as in the case described.

2 E – Ovarian carcinoma

Ovarian carcinoma is responsible for the fourth highest number of cancer deaths in women in the UK. Most of the cancers are of epithelial origin, and the peak incidence occurs in women aged 50–70 years. The aetiology is unknown but genetic factors are increasingly recognised as being important (*BRCA1*). In addition, 'incessant ovulation' appears important as nulliparity, early menarche and a late menopause are frequently associated with its development, whereas use of the contraceptive pill, which inhibits ovulation, affords protection. Most epithelial tumours are advanced at presentation, having spread beyond the pelvis, because of the insidious nature of symptoms and signs. Consequently, the overall 5-year survival rate is less than 25%. Presenting symptoms are frequently vague and non-specific. Abdominal distension and pain (secondary to peritoneal seeding and ascites formation: stage III), weight loss, anorexia, and occasionally a hard-irregular mass arising in the pelvis are the commonest symptoms. Pleural effusion with positive cytology confirms distant spread of disease (stage IV). Surgery is the mainstay of both diagnosis and treatment of ovarian cancer and involves debulking of tumour wherever possible.

3 G – Renal cell carcinoma

Renal cell carcinoma arises from the cells of the proximal convoluted tubule. It commonly affects individuals in their sixth or seventh decade, and is twice as common in men. It presents commonly with one or more of the classic triad: haematuria, loin pain and palpable mass (all present in this case).

INDEX

Note to reader: Entries are indexed by question number, not by page number.